DEVELOPING SPEED

National Strength and Conditioning Association

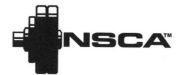

Ian Jeffreys

EDITOR

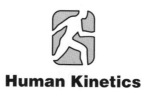

Human Kinetics

Library of Congress Cataloging-in-Publication Data

Developing speed / National Strength & Conditioning Association (U.S.) ; Ian Jeffreys, editor.
    pages cm -- (Sport performance series)
    Includes bibliographical references and index.
    1. Physical education and training. 2. Athletes--Training of. 3. Physical fitness--Physiological aspects. 4. Muscle strength. 5. Speed. I. Jeffreys, Ian. II. National Strength & Conditioning Association (U.S.)
    GV711.5.D477 2013
    613.7'11--dc23
                                      2013003156

ISBN-10: 0-7360-8328-6 (print)
ISBN-13: 978-0-7360-8328-7 (print)

This publication is written and published to provide accurate and authoritative information relevant to the subject matter presented. It is published and sold with the understanding that the author and publisher are not engaged in rendering legal, medical, or other professional services by reason of their authorship or publication of this work. If medical or other expert assistance is required, the services of a competent professional person should be sought.

Assistant Acquisitions Editor: Justin Klug; **Developmental Editor:** Heather Healy; **Assistant Editors:** Claire Marty and Tyler Wolpert; **Copyeditor:** Annette Pierce; **Indexer:** Nan N. Badgett; **Permissions Manager:** Martha Gullo; **Graphic Designer:** Joe Buck; **Graphic Artist:** Tara Welsch; **Cover Designer:** Keith Blomberg; **Photograph (cover):** © Bob Thomas/iStockphoto; **Photographs (interior):** © Human Kinetics unless otherwise noted; **Photo Asset Manager:** Laura Fitch; **Visual Production Assistant:** Joyce Brumfield; **Photo Production Manager:** Jason Allen; **Art Manager:** Kelly Hendren; **Associate Art Manager:** Alan L. Wilborn; **Illustrations:** © Human Kinetics, unless otherwise noted; **Printer:** Versa Press

We thank the National Strength and Conditioning Association in Colorado Springs, Colorado, and the High School of St. Thomas More in Champaign, Illinois, for assistance in providing the location for the photo shoot for this book.

Human Kinetics books are available at special discounts for bulk purchase. Special editions or book excerpts can also be created to specification. For details, contact the Special Sales Manager at Human Kinetics.

Printed in the United States of America   10 9 8 7 6 5 4 3 2 1

The paper in this book is certified under a sustainable forestry program.

Human Kinetics
Website: www.HumanKinetics.com

United States: Human Kinetics
P.O. Box 5076
Champaign, IL 61825-5076
800-747-4457
e-mail: humank@hkusa.com

Canada: Human Kinetics
475 Devonshire Road Unit 100
Windsor, ON N8Y 2L5
800-465-7301 (in Canada only)
e-mail: info@hkcanada.com

Europe: Human Kinetics
107 Bradford Road
Stanningley
Leeds LS28 6AT, United Kingdom
+44 (0) 113 255 5665
e-mail: hk@hkeurope.com

Australia: Human Kinetics
57A Price Avenue
Lower Mitcham, South Australia 5062
08 8372 0999
e-mail: info@hkaustralia.com

New Zealand: Human Kinetics
P.O. Box 80
Torrens Park, South Australia 5062
0800 222 062
e-mail: info@hknewzealand.com

E4820

DEVELOPING SPEED

Contents

Introduction

Ask athletes what aspect of performance they would like to improve the most and their answer normally is sprint speed. This is because speed is often the most important factor in differentiating between being a great athlete and being a good athlete. The striker in soccer beating the defender to the ball and scoring the winning goal, the tennis player running down a crosscourt shot before playing a winner down the line, or the wide receiver outrunning the defense for a game-winning touchdown are all examples of the importance of speed in sport. Given this importance, it is no surprise that tests of running speed play a large role in evaluation programs for sport. Similarly, athletes with great speed are highly sought out in a variety of sports.

For a long time, speed was viewed as a genetic trait that could not be improved. However, this belief has been found to be false, and although genetics play a role in determining the top speed an athlete can reach, speed is a trainable component. Athletes can improve running speed if they follow a well-designed and scientifically based training program. This book provides athletes and coaches with the tools to improve speed. The book gathers some of the world's leading authorities in speed development and the application of speed training to specific sports. This information allows coaches and athletes to develop speed training programs that will maximize sport-specific speed.

This book provides a combination of background knowledge and practical application. Rather than containing just a variety of drills, the book also offers information to help coaches and athletes understand how speed training works and why certain drills and exercises are included. This allows coaches and athletes to make informed decisions about training and to adapt it to their program to suit their specific needs. This background information helps coaches and athletes understand what each exercise is meant to accomplish and guides them toward selecting exercises focused on the specific technical flaws that need to be corrected.

Another critical aspect of the book is the application of speed training to sport. While track and field speed training models emphasize general speed development, the crucial element in developing speed for sport is how well the improvement transfers to sport performance itself. As a result, a large proportion of the book is dedicated to developing speed in sport-specific situations. This includes a section on constructing general speed programs followed by sections on developing speed for specific sports.

Key to Diagrams

▲ Cone

∿ Hurdle

▯ Pole

⟶ Sprint or player movement

- - -▸ Side shuffle

·········▸ Backpedal

∿∿∿▸ Forward skate

∿∿▸ Backward skate

- - - ▸ Path of hit or pass

∿∿∿▸ Dribble

X Athlete's starting position, defensive player, or any player

O Offensive player

C Coach

The Nature of Speed

Ian Jeffreys

It is often said in sporting circles that speed kills. This emphasizes how speed has long been recognized as a major component of superior performance in many sports. The extensive use of speed tests to identify talent and monitor performance in most sports further attests to the importance of speed in performance. Similarly, the high value placed on fast athletes further emphasizes speed's value to high-level performance. Whereas speed once was seen as largely a genetic trait that could not be affected greatly by training, today we recognize that a well-structured and scientifically sound training program can improve speed. Such a program is outlined in this book and provides a tried and trusted formula for enhancing running speed.

Because speed can be enhanced through a scientifically sound program, athletes and coaches must develop a fundamental knowledge of the factors that contribute to speed in order to maximize the benefits of training. This chapter provides a general knowledge of the science behind effective speed performance, enabling coaches and athletes to make informed decisions as they integrate the information into their own training. Armed with this knowledge, coaches and athletes are able to select appropriate elements from the book and apply them to their own training, whatever their sport and whatever their ability. In understanding the scientific concepts of training, they also are able to adapt practices to provide the ideal training environment for any situation.

DEFINING SPEED

Any discussion on improving running speed must start with an examination of what speed is. In scientific terms, speed equals distance divided by time and is normally measured in meters per second. However, in performance terms, it is useful to look at speed as the time taken to cover a given distance. Indeed, most performance is measured by the time taken to cover a specific distance rather than an actual measure of speed. This subtle difference helps in setting up sport-specific speed development programs.

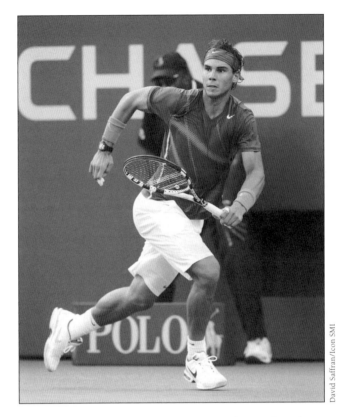

David Saffran/Icon SMI

Rafael Nadal has excellent gamespeed, running the width of the court in a few seconds to return a shot.

Although basic running speed is an important aspect of performance in many sports, equally important is the ability to express this in the context of the sport: the concept of *gamespeed*. Gamespeed is the application of speed in a sport specific context, which maximizes sport performance. Aspects such as the typical distances covered, the direction of the distances, the signals that trigger movement, and the actions that will be carried out when an athlete reaches a given point vary from sport to sport and need to be taken into account when designing sport-specific speed development programs. These aspects, together with a system to evaluate sport speed requirements, are covered in chapter 5. Applying the system to specific sports is covered in chapter 6.

POTENTIAL FOR AND LIMITS OF SPEED DEVELOPMENT

Although speed can be improved, it is inaccurate to suggest that everyone has the capacity to become a sprint champion. A genetic ceiling exists for the top speed an athlete can reach, therefore limiting the ability of the vast majority of people to become an Olympic 100-meter champion. However, while this ceiling exists, it is likely that few people actually reach their ceiling. This is clearly demonstrated by the improvements that elite sprinters make throughout their careers. If top sprinters, with their training aimed specifically at speed development, do not always reach their full genetic potential, then clearly, the likelihood of athletes involved in other sports reaching their speed ceiling is much lower. Therefore, a majority of athletes have a great potential for improving speed, and speed development programs are fundamental to any total performance enhancement program. It is hoped that as speed training methods improve and are used by more and more athletes, more people will approach their ceiling and reach their full speed potential.

The principal genetic limits to performance are the type of muscle fiber, their activation, and the athlete's body type and structure. Great sprinters have a preponderance of fast-twitch muscle fibers. Fast-twitch fibers have a higher force-producing capacity and a higher speed of contraction but are less resistant to fatigue than slow-twitch fibers. Clearly, the higher the percentage of fast-twitch fibers an athlete has, the greater the capacity for speed.

This is further emphasized by the fact that there are two major types of fast-twitch fibers: Type IIa and Type IIx. Type IIx fibers demonstrate the greatest force-production capacity and contraction speed but exhibit very limited endurance. Type IIa fibers still have a high force capacity and speed of contraction, although not as high as Type IIx fibers, but have a greater endurance capacity than Type IIx. Elite sprinters have a high overall percentage of Type II fibers and also a high percentage of Type IIx fibers.

While the proportion of an athlete's muscle fiber types is predominantly set at birth, training can affect their characteristics and how they are activated. Prolonged endurance training for example can lead to Type IIx fibers taking on the characteristics of Type IIa fibers and to Type IIa fibers taking on the characteristics of Type I. Both of these effects reduce the force capacity of the muscle, especially in relation to the rate at which force can be applied. Additionally, excessive periods of resistance training, especially where slow movements are stressed, can lead to a change in fiber characteristics between Type IIx and Type IIa.

Also important is how effective an athlete is at recruiting the Type II muscle fibers (especially Type IIx). Untrained athletes typically recruit only a limited proportion of Type IIx muscle fibers, and training with high loads or high speeds or both is required to develop the capacity to recruit a high proportion of Type IIx fibers. Therefore, a speed development program needs to include resistance training that uses high loads and explosive movement.

Another important genetic factor in speed development is each athlete's body structure. Lever lengths (length of arms and legs) greatly determine the capacity to move rapidly, and the length of these levers is determined by both bone length and the point at which the muscles insert into the bone. This means that some bodies are designed ideally to move rapidly while others are not. Again this factor is genetically limited.

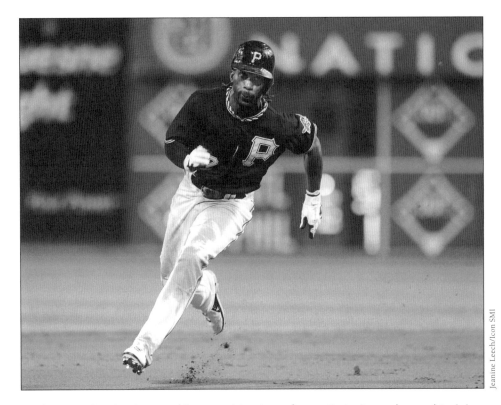

Jeanine Leech/Icon SMI

Andrew McCutchen's speed is a combination of genetic traits and speed training.

Although genetic limits provide a theoretical ceiling for speed capacity, the focus of a speed development program is improvement of this capacity and especially how it relates to sport performance. It is important, therefore, to look at the aspects of speed that can be improved. This requires an examination of the nature of running speed and identifying the elements that can be enhanced through training. In this way, athletes and coaches can focus on the elements they can adapt, which then become the focus of a speed improvement program.

While the focus of this book is how to develop sport-specific speed, little research has been conducted into how speed is expressed directly in sport settings. However, a large body of work exists in track and field and in scientifically based measurements of linear speed. For this reason, we will examine sprinting, with the aim of developing generalizations we can apply to speed development in sport. The aim of sprinting is to move horizontally from one point to another as rapidly as possible. Therefore, generating horizontal velocity is vital. This requires generating an impulse (measured as the force applied multiplied by the duration of the force application) to move the body horizontally and the ability to maximize the effectiveness of this movement.

Sprinting can be viewed in two ways. In one train of thought, sprinting is a finely coordinated motor skill, emphasizing finely tuned movements. In another view, sprinting is a ballistic activity, with the body driven forward as a projectile in a series of muscular efforts. While these views may appear diametrically opposed, they are both true. Sprinting depends on skilled movements, and it also depends on ballistic forces. Therefore, training for speed is multidimensional and must involve a range of activities that address all of the factors that contribute to speed. One of the greatest skills in developing speed is choosing the activities that best meet the needs of an athlete at a given time and to coordinate these into an effective training program.

DETERMINANTS OF RUNNING SPEED

Two factors that determine running speed are stride cadence and stride length. Stride cadence refers to the number of strides taken per second, and stride length refers to the distance traveled by each stride. The product of these factors gives a mathematically accurate description of running speed. Traditional thinking has suggested that if one of these can be improved with the other remaining constant, running speed will increase. Therefore, the focus of speed training has been on improving stride cadence, improving stride length, or improving both. However, recent research suggests that while improving these factors plays a role in determining running speed, they may provide the coach limited tools when developing speed training programs.

In particular, the concept of stride length, traditionally measured as the distance between each successive foot contact, can be problematic. Too much focus on artificially lengthening an athlete's stride can result in placing the foot ahead of the athlete's center of mass. This position compromises the athlete's ability to generate force and ultimately slows running speed. Instead, an effective stride length should be the focus. This is the distance traveled by the athlete's center of gravity per stride. An effective stride length is generated by applying a force into the ground (pushing off the ground) and propelling the athlete forward rather than reaching forward with the legs in an attempt to pull the athlete forward. The force producing capacities of the athlete are fundamental to achieving optimal stride and length and maximal speed.

Stride cadence is a function of contact time (the time spent on the ground with each stride) and flight time (the time spent in the air on each stride). Research has shown little variation in flight time between runners of different speeds, and the greatest variations in cadence are a result of differences in ground contact time (Weyand et al. 2000). Therefore, efforts to improve stride cadence should focus on shortening ground-contact times rather than focusing on cycling the legs faster.

Stride length is largely a function of the impulse and velocity generated at toe-off. The velocity of the athlete's center of gravity, which is a key factor in dictating stride length, does not alter between successive steps. Like impulse, it is generated during the time the athlete's foot is in contact with the ground (the stance phase). Therefore, efforts to enhance stride length by technical means during the flight phase, the time the body is not in contact with the ground, are limited and should instead focus on generating impulse and velocity during the time the athlete is in contact with the ground.

The discussion of stride length and stride cadence requires an analysis of the phases of a running stride. Each running stride can be divided into two components: a stance phase and a flight phase. These phases are outlined in figure 1.1. The stance phase occurs when the athlete's foot is on the ground

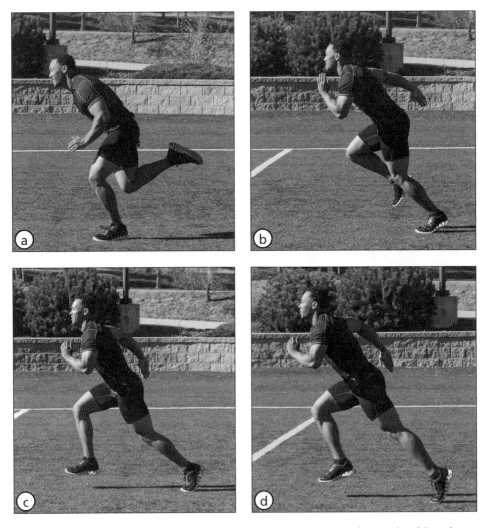

Figure 1.1 Running stride consists of a three-part stance phase: the *(a)* early stance, *(b)* midstance, and *(c)* late stance, followed by *(d)* the flight phase.

and consists of the time between the initial contact with the ground and the subsequent toe-off.

The stance phase can be further divided into an early stance, a midstance, and a late stance. During the early stance, when the foot makes contact with the ground, the athlete's body absorbs the landing forces, which can vary from two and a half to five times the bodyweight, depending on the speed and distance of a sprint. The leg muscles absorb the landing forces through eccentric contraction, which lengthens the muscles. This has the potential to cause significant braking forces unless the athlete has the strength capacities and required muscle stiffness to effectively repel this force. During this phase, the athlete can develop elastic energy, which is beneficial in later stages. During the midstance, the athlete switches from absorbing force to exerting a concentric force, which shortens the muscles and generates maximal vertical force. The elastic energy generated in the early stance can contribute to the force produced through the mid and late stance. In late stance, the body accelerates forward as a result of the concentric forces generated.

The flight phase is the period between toe-off and the next foot contact (see figure 1.2). During this phase the athlete makes no contact with the ground, so in essence is in flight. Velocity during the flight phase cannot be increased, and the athlete must cycle the leg in preparation for the next footfall. An inability to cycle the leg effectively results in suboptimal ground contact on the next stance phase, and therefore limits speed expression. Because athletes can propel themselves forward only when their foot is in contact with the ground, the stance phase should be the main focus of speed enhancement programs.

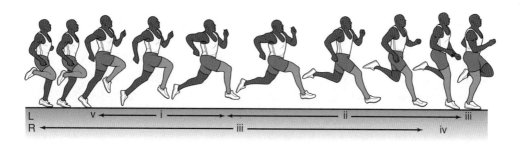

Figure 1.2 Sprinting technique at maximum velocity. In this illustration, the left and right legs show the phases of the running stride: (i) early flight, (ii) midflight, (iii) late flight, (iv) early stance, and (v) late stance.

Adapted, by permission, from G. Schmolinsky, 2000, *Track and field: The East German textbook of athletics* (Toronto: Sport Books), 122-123.

BIOMECHANICS OF SPEED

We have discussed how horizontal propulsion is generated during the stance phase. Now we will look at the rules governing motion and force production. Biomechanics is the study of forces and their effects on living systems (McGinnis 2005), and because forces determine motion, a fundamental understanding of the biomechanical principles that affect speed can assist coaches and athletes in developing running speed.

Speed clearly involves motion, and so to maximize its effectiveness, speed training should be guided by the scientific principles of motion. In 1687, renowned British scientist Sir Isaac Newton published his famous book, commonly referred to as *Principia*. Published in Latin, the language of science at that time, the book contained his three laws of motion, the fundamentals of which still hold true today and that contribute greatly to understanding the training concepts for speed development. Newton's three laws of motion—the law of inertia, the law of acceleration, and the law of action and reaction—translated into English read as follows:

▶ **Law 1—Law of inertia.** Every body continues in its state of rest or of uniform motion in a straight line unless it is compelled to change that state by forces impressed upon it.

▶ **Law 2—Law of acceleration.** The change of motion of an object is proportional to the force impressed and is made in the direction of the straight line in which the force is impressed.

▶ **Law 3—Law of action and reaction.** To every action there is always an opposite and equal reaction or the mutual actions of two bodies upon each other are always equal and directed to contrary parts.

At first, these may appear to be overly scientific and have little importance to speed training. However, when examined more closely and worded more simply, they play a vital role in planning effective speed training. An understanding of these rules, together with the application of their impact will help coaches and athletes make informed decisions in many elements of speed development.

Law 1 states that any time motion needs to be started or changed, a force must be applied. In terms of running speed, this force comes from within the body in the form of a muscular action, and so, every time an athlete wants to start moving or change the motion (for example increase speed, decrease speed, or change direction), the athlete needs to apply a force. Without the application of force, motion cannot be initiated or changed. A change in the direction or quantity of motion is termed acceleration and so any acceleration requires the application of a force.

This then leads to the second law, where the rate of change of motion (acceleration) is proportional to the amount of force applied. This is a cause-and-effect relationship, where force directly causes acceleration. This is indeed one of the most important messages an athlete or coach needs to take onboard when designing a speed training program: The rate of acceleration depends on the force applied. The second law of motion is summarized by the following equation:

$$Force = Mass \times Acceleration$$

In terms of running, mass can be assumed to be constant; therefore, acceleration is directly dependent on, and proportional to, the force applied. The ability to produce force effectively and rapidly is essential. The amount of force required, though, depends on the athletic task or movement to be performed. Therefore, training must be specific to each task to develop a range of movement patterns.

This also brings up another important element for long-term speed development: the role of mass, or the athlete's weight. Increased mass requires greater force to achieve the acceleration. Therefore, when athletes use resistance training they must make sure an increase in body weight coincides with an increase in strength. Increasing muscle size without also increasing the ability to produce force does nothing to improve the ability to accelerate. Strength training for speed development should focus on increasing force-producing capacity not on increasing muscle size.

The key message from the third law—for every action there is an equal and opposite reaction—is illustrated when running forces are applied into the ground, which then pushes the athlete upward and forward with an equal and opposite force. This brings into focus the importance of the direction of the application of force as well as its quantity. Force needs to be applied in a direction opposite to the intended direction of motion. Speed, therefore, is maximized when both the quantity and direction of the force are optimal.

Taking all of these laws together, it can be seen that ground forces largely determine acceleration and running speed. Thus, improving the application of ground forces needs to be a major focus of any speed training program.

ACCELERATION VS. MAXIMUM SPEED

Acceleration and maximum speed are terms used in speed development programs, and when developing a program, it is vital to differentiate between them. This allows coaches to target their training to the capacity most important in their own sport. Acceleration is the rate of change of velocity, or how quickly an athlete can increase the velocity of the motion. Maximum speed is the highest rate of speed an athlete can attain.

Acceleration refers to velocity, and because velocity has both a magnitude and direction associated with it, acceleration changes when athletes change the magnitude of their motion (how fast they are running), the direction of their motion, or both. In terms of running, anytime the body starts, speeds up, or changes direction, it is accelerating. Given the number of direction changes in most sports, together with the number of times the rate of velocity needs to change, then clearly acceleration plays a crucial role in speed performance in sport. This is further emphasized by the fact that elite sprinters have been shown to take up to 60 meters to reach top speed, and while this distance is normally shorter for field sport athletes, it still takes a considerable distance for most athletes to reach their maximum speed. Given the typical distances run in sport and the limits of court dimension in other sports, such as tennis and basketball, acceleration may play a more important role than maximum speed in these sports.

However, as chapter 2 demonstrates, maximum speed still plays an important role in sport because athletes can still reach a high proportion of their maximal speed in a relatively short distance. Figures from the International Associations of Athletics Federations have shown that during his 100 meter final in the Beijing Olympics, Usain Bolt achieved 73 percent of his maximum velocity at 10 meters, 85 percent at 20 meters, 93 percent at 30 meters, and 96 percent at 40 meters. He attained maximum speed at 60 meters. Therefore, developing maximum

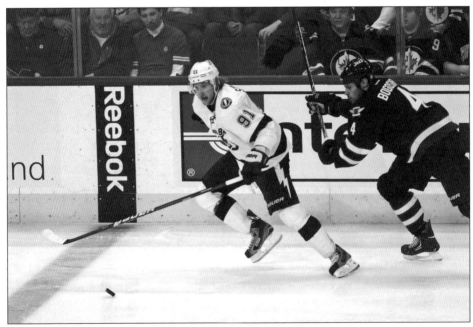

Terry Lee/Icon SMI

While attaining maximal speed is limited by the size of the hockey rink, Steven Stamkos uses his acceleration speed to out-maneuver his opponent.

speed should still be included in the training for most sports, but the relative importance of the two should dictate the time spent on each.

While acceleration and maximum speed are two different qualities, acceleration is the process by which an athlete attempts to move toward maximum speed. For this reason, the process of acceleration goes through distinct phases. In the initial phase, an athlete's velocity is low, and therefore the capacity to increase velocity is great. This is the pure acceleration phase, often referred to in track sprinting as the drive phase. However, as distance increases, athletes approach speeds far closer to their maximum, and this is the transition acceleration phase. For example, in the Usain Bolt figures listed earlier, at 30 meters Bolt had attained 93 percent of his maximum velocity, while at 10 meters he had only attained 73 percent. Thus, as distance increases, the capacity for further acceleration decreases. Similarly, the key technical features of acceleration differ at these stages.

GRAVITY AND FORCE APPLICATION

In addition to the laws of motion, Newton's scientific legacy has had another important impact on speed development: the law of gravity. Whatever the sport, athletes are subject to a gravitational force that causes acceleration toward the earth at a rate of 9.8 meters per second per second. As we have discussed, sprinting is concerned with maximizing horizontal impulse. However, sprinters also need to ensure that they exert sufficient vertical force to overcome gravity and create sufficient time to reposition their legs effectively for the successive stride.

Therefore, the ideal force vector is one in which sufficient vertical force is applied to enable leg repositioning, with the remainder applied horizontally to provide propulsion. In reality, it is impossible to independently alter the horizontal and vertical aspect of the resultant force vector. The direction of the net force, therefore, depends on body position, the overall force the athlete applies, and the muscles activated.

Ground Contact Time

Because the application of force is fundamental to running speed, and because force can only be applied when the foot is on the ground, we will examine the ground contact times during pure acceleration, transition acceleration, and maximum speed. Ground contact times are at their greatest during pure acceleration (approximately .2 second), decrease through transition acceleration (.12 second in late transition), and decrease to .09 to .10 at maximum speed. This has important consequences for force-producing capacity. Because impulse is the force applied multiplied by the duration of force application, when ground contact time decreases, the net impulse also decreases. Therefore, during acceleration, greater ground contact times allow for greater impulse, so force can be directed both vertically and horizontally.

However, as speed increases and ground contact time decreases, more force is needed vertically to overcome the force of gravity, and less is available for horizontal propulsion. There comes a point at which ground contact time is so short that all of the force equals what is required to overcome gravity, and at that point, no additional force can be directed toward horizontal propulsion. At this point the athlete can no longer accelerate and has attained maximal velocity.

As mentioned previously, stride length and stride cadence are factors that affect running speed. Overall stride cadence is related closely to ground contact times, and stride length is related to the impulse produced during ground contact. Thus, a key element of speed may be the ability to produce more force in a shorter time. Faster sprinters consistently demonstrate shorter ground contact times than slower sprinters. This indicates their ability to exert force rapidly. This requires the development of appropriate strength and power characteristics, including optimal stiffness and eccentric and concentric force capacity.

Part of a sprinters' ability to shorten ground contact times may be caused by their ability to terminate the stance phase earlier, allowing them to cycle the leg through as efficiently as possible. This earlier termination of the stance phase has been shown in both acceleration and maximum-speed running. This appears to be achieved by the initiation of hip flexion before the completion of the stance. Additionally, it requires high levels of stiffness in the knee and ankle to allow for the rapid absorption of the eccentric landing forces, the activation of the stretch-shortening cycle (SSC), and subsequent concentric force production.

Although athletes apply impulses during the stance phase, the flight phase also plays an important preparatory role for effective force production. At high velocities, athletes must reposition the swing leg rapidly in order to prepare for the next stance phase. This becomes increasingly important as ground contact times decrease and the athletes have to apply predominantly vertical forces to overcome gravity. This rapid cycling action requires a triple flexion of the hip, knee, and ankle, which results in shortening the lever and allowing a rapid recovery cycle (cycling the leg through to the next stance phase). This ability needs to be developed through appropriate technical development.

Directional Force Application

Because the horizontal and vertical aspects of force cannot be split, the athlete needs to generate forces that reflect the relative importance of each. One of the major ways to do this is through posture. The changes in posture during a sprint are dictated by the direction that the force needs to be applied. In the early phases of a sprint there is little momentum, and so an athlete needs to generate forward momentum. This requires that force be applied horizontally and vertically to overcome the influence of gravity. In the initial acceleration, horizontal and vertical forces are equally distributed, resulting in a forward lean at a 45-degree angle (see figure 1.3). At this time, ideal running technique involves a pistonlike action, enabling the generation of the forces needed to drive horizontally and vertically. Therefore, the technical acceleration exercises in chapter 3 develop this pistonlike action.

However, as athletes approach top speed, they have produced considerable horizontal momentum, and the major requirement is to overcome gravity in order to allow for an effective leg cycle. In this situation, the resultant forces are predominantly vertical (see figure 1.4). This line of force application and the application of optimal posture are explored further in chapter 2. Similarly, the technical exercises for maximum speed in chapter 3 are aimed at developing this vertical technique and rapid cycling action of the leg.

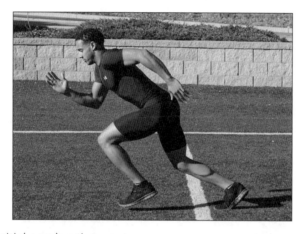

Figure 1.3 Initial acceleration posture.

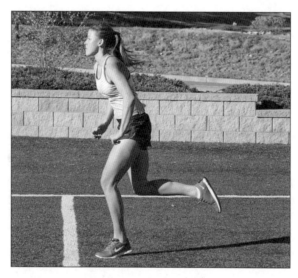

Figure 1.4 Maximal speed posture.

Optimizing Force Development

Newton's laws clearly emphasize the role of force in optimizing acceleration and maximum speed. Next we look at ways to optimize an athlete's capacity to develop force. (This book cannot discuss all aspects of force production. More details on this can be found in books specifically on strength and power development.)

In running, force can be applied only when the foot is on the ground and thus, always functions under a time restriction. This is critical when analyzing force requirements for developing running speed. The force–velocity relationship states that high forces require a relatively large amount of time to be applied, and when time is restricted, maximum force can never be achieved. In this way, it is not always an athlete's maximum-force capacity that determines running speed but rather how much force can be applied in a given time. Thus, speed depends on a capacity known as the rate of force development.

The length of ground contact time is greatest in the initial phases of acceleration (approximately .2 second; refer to figure 1.3 and see figure 1.5) and gradually decreases until at maximum speed (about .1 second; refer to figures 1.2 and 1.4). In this way, maximum force capacity has the biggest impact on initial acceleration, while the rate of force development together with the ability to store and use elastic energy (the stretch-shortening cycle) play an increasingly important role as the distance of the run increases.

The development of maximum force, the rate of force development, and the development of the stretch-shortening cycle require different strength training interventions, and all of these must be addressed when designing a speed development program. However, the fact that all of these elements can be improved means that the majority of athletes have a great capacity to improve running speed.

During a sprint, forces are developed initially through the hips, then the knee joint, and finally through the ankle joint. This movement is known as triple extension. Therefore, activities that maximize the triple extension abilities of

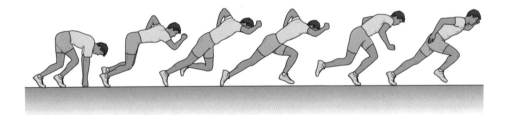

Figure 1.5 Ground contact time is greatest during acceleration.

Adapted, by permission, from G. Schmolinsky, 2000, *Track and field: The East German textbook of athletics* (Toronto: Sport Books).

the athlete should play a large role in the training to enhance speed and acceleration. Exercises such as the squat, Olympic lifts, and hip extension exercises such as the Romanian deadlift should form the basis of a strength and power program for speed enhancement.

As speed increases, the athlete is required initially to absorb landing forces and then to repel these forces, essentially rebounding off the ground. During running, the initial ground contact results in a braking force, and the athlete's strength largely determines how well these forces are absorbed. The size of the braking force relates to the phase of the sprint and the speed of the athlete. This is emphasized by the fact that during a sprint, ground and muscle support forces can exceed bodyweight by two and a half to five times, with the value increasing with increased speed.

The body therefore needs to overcome these braking forces and produce propulsive forces to continue accelerating or to maintain maximum speed. These propulsive forces are a combination of voluntary concentric forces and reflexive, SSC-based forces. The concentric portion is greatest in early acceleration, while the SSC-based forces dominate at higher speeds. In this way, the leg muscles act in a springlike fashion. This springlike quality is maximized with greater stiffness, and increased stability of the knee and ankle can optimize both reflexive force production and ground contact times. Plyometric exercises can enhance this springlike quality through enhancing an athlete's stretch shortening cycle capacities.

So far, our discussion of the strength and power program has focused on the lower body and the generation of ground forces. However, the core and upper body also contribute to maximizing ground forces and, hence, effective running speed. The total force applied to the ground is enhanced by an effective arm action in which the arm drives downward and backward. Therefore, increased force capacity in this action can assist in net force production at the ground. Similarly, a stable and strong core can optimize force development, force transfer, and force application. This allows forces to be transferred through the body and into the ground without the loss of energy or force through unnecessary compensatory movements of the trunk. This emphasizes the importance of posture on speed, and the development of appropriate posture and postural control are areas of focus in chapter 2.

SKILLED NATURE OF SPEED

Undoubtedly, ground forces play a major role in speed development and explain the view of sprinting as a series of ballistic strides. However, developing the athlete's capacity to produce force should be seen as just one part of the speed equation. It is vital that force capacities transfer into enhanced ground reaction forces and enhanced speed. However, although force is important, sprinters cannot be built solely in the weight room. Instead, they need to ensure that the gains made in the weight room transfer onto the field.

Here the view of speed as a coordinated motor action is important. Running speed and acceleration are skills and need to be trained in the same manner as other skills. In this way the coordinative elements of speed assume an important role. Athletes need to learn how to assume effective postures and how to use and coordinate arm and leg actions to maximize ground force and stride cadence and, thus, maximize running speed and acceleration. Effective technique maximizes stride effectiveness through appropriate lever alignments and maximal efficiency, thus conserving energy. (See chapter 2 for key technical areas to address.)

PROCESS OF SKILL DEVELOPMENT

All athletes learn skills through three stages: the motor (cognitive) stage, the associative stage, and the autonomous stage. Although running may seem a natural ability, a look at typical running actions on any playground or sport field demonstrates that it is anything but. Effective running actions need to be taught and practiced repeatedly if they are to become engrained in the athlete. Chapters 2 and 3 focus on the development of running actions. Chapter 2 outlines the technical requirements of running, and chapter 3 looks at exercises to develop technique.

To maximize the productivity of an exercise or practice, it is important to understand the characteristics and requirements of the athletes in each of the phases. In this way, training sessions and programs become learning opportunities in which technique is developed and constantly honed until it becomes a skilled act that can stand up under pressure.

In the motor phase, athletes are learning the skill. Here, their movements are often uncoordinated, jerky, and inconsistent. Their focus, therefore, needs to be almost totally on the task at hand. The challenge of the exercise should be limited, focusing on single tasks. Because the movements are unstable, they often break down, so a challenge such as a competitive run should be closely monitored and limited so it doesn't interfere with learning the skill.

Similarly, exercises to develop technique should emphasize the quality of performance and the speed of performance to ensure the development of appropriate technique. Coaches should limit the technical complexity of their feedback at this time. Guidelines for coaching athletes in the cognitive stage (Jeffreys 2007) are summarized in table 1.1.

In the associative phase, an athlete's performance shows much more coordination and consistency. At this time, exercises can be challenging in terms of their complexity, speed, and the level of competition. This progression should develop through the stage and should be guided by the athlete's performance. A coach should not worry about regressing an exercise if performance breaks

Table 1.1 Guidelines for Coaching at Each Stage of Motor Development

Motor (cognitive) stage	Associative stage	Autonomous stage
Focus on developing technique.	Continue to hone technique while increasing challenges.	Develop the ability to maintain technique in gamelike situations.
Focus largely on general speed capabilities.	Continue to develop general capacities and also start to apply these to game conditions.	Focus on the application of speed while continuing to present general work to ensure these capacities are maintained.
Use selective drills to develop targeted technical capacities where required (e.g., arm-action drills, wall drills).	Continue to use drills and supplement them with more applied work.	Focus on applied work, with drills used in warm-ups and other situations to maintain technical capacities.
Focus on a few selective movements per session.	Increase the variety of exercises per session.	Provide a high degree of variation within and between sessions.
Use a great deal of noncompetitive work to focus on technique.	Add more competitive work, but not at the expense of technique.	Practice much of the work in competitive situations.
Practice in a nonfatigued state.	Practice in a nonfatigued state.	Practice predominantly in a nonfatigued state, but introduce challenges to develop the ability to run at speed under pressure.
Enhance learning through the use of demonstrations and develop key technical cues.	Use the key cues to reinforce technique as appropriate. Use demonstrations as required.	Use key cues to reinforce technique where breakdowns occur.
Use a great deal of simple feedback.	Reduce the quantity of feedback, but increase its precision.	Give feedback infrequently, and make sure it is precise.

Reprinted, by permission, from I. Jeffreys, 2007, *Total soccer fitness* (Monterey, CA: Coaches Choice).

down. As an athlete's movements become more automated, more challenging exercises can be introduced, which requires focus on both speed of performance and external factors such as reacting to different stimuli. See table 1.1 for guidelines for coaching at the associative stage (Jeffreys 2007).

After considerable practice, some athletes will enter the autonomous stage, where movement patterns are of high quality and are consistent. At the autonomous stage, movement patterns are well developed, and the athletes' aim is to perfect these patterns while also ensuring that they can use them effectively and consistently in intense sport-specific environments. This stage sees a predominance of high-intensity, highly complex drills. Coaching input is less frequent but more detailed and includes precise feedback. Guidelines for coaching at the autonomous phase are summarized in table 1.1. (Jeffreys 2007).

KEY ELEMENTS OF SPEED TRAINING

This chapter has demonstrated that speed relies on both motor skill development and the development of physical capacities to produce effective ground-reaction forces. For these reasons, a speed development program should include three key elements:

▶ **Development of physical capacities.** An effective speed development program must develop an athlete's force production capacity in the musculature involved in sprinting. Each of the following is likely to play an important role in determining running speed:

- Maximal force capacity
- Rate of force development
- Stretch-shortening cycle ability

▶ **Technical development.** Development of sound running technique helps ensure that athletes can use their physical capacities to enhance their speed. Technical training targets areas of deficiency in the running action. This form of training starts with an analysis of performance and then addresses areas of deficiency such as arm action, leg action, and so on.

▶ **Application of speed.** The development of technique and the development of physical capacities are of no benefit unless they enhance running speed in the sport-specific context. Thus, the critical question is how to effectively transfer them to enhance gamespeed. This transfer requires an athlete to perform high-quality, sport-specific bursts of speed. While this may seem obvious, much field sport training neglects frequent high-speed running. Thus, a speed improvement program must involve speed application and address all of the elements that affect performance in a particular sport, such as initial acceleration, transition acceleration, and maximum speed. Later chapters in the book outline methods of directly applying speed in sport-specific contexts.

These three elements should be integrated into a speed development program. The omission of any of these will result in less than optimal results. These elements also should be tailored to the individual athlete's characteristics. Some athletes use great technique but lack the physical capacities to maximize this technique. Others may possess excellent physical capacities but lack the required technique to optimize them. Therefore, the focus of specific elements is different for each athlete. No speed development program will be universally optimal, so coaches need to adjust programs in response to these differences. Undoubtedly, the more knowledge a coach or athlete has regarding the scientific principles of program design, the more effectively they will be able to adapt programs to their specific needs.

CHAPTER 2

Technical Models of Speed

Jeremy Sheppard

As covered in chapter 1, speed is not a single entity, so to best understand a sprint effort, view it in several phases: acceleration (including pure acceleration and transition acceleration), maximum speed, and deceleration. These phases occur during a typical track sprint but also occur during the vast majority of sports. Their relative importance depends on the specific requirements of the sport involved. These phases of sprinting are not separate events, and, generally, a fluid transition takes place between them. However, unique characteristics are inherent in each and form the basis of the technical development (see chapter 3). Understanding the aspects of the sprint enables the coach and athlete to increase their awareness of the biomechanics involved in sprinting, refine technique, and improve performance.

In regards to the technical models of sprinting, there is debate about the application of track sprinting principles to running in field and court sports such as American football (as well as rugby and Australian rules football), soccer, basketball, tennis, and so on. This debate seems to involve two primary discussion points:

1. The technical differences that may exist between sprinting in track (a known, straight sprint) and sprinting in field and court sports

2. The role of maximum speed in field and court sports

This chapter addresses these points; however, track models can provide a frame of reference around which to construct effective technique applicable across many sports.

SPRINTING IN FIELD AND COURT SPORTS

While track sprinting is a closed skill, athletes in field and court sports require reactive agility. Athletes must accelerate, decelerate, and change direction in a constantly changing environment, performing skills within the context of the game. Furthermore, athletes in field and court sports need to scan a broader area and use different postures to aid in collisions, allow for deception against an opponent, or to prepare for likely direction changes (Sayers 2000). These requirements result in technical differences between sprinting in a field or court sport and sprinting the 100 meters (Sayers 2000, Gambetta 1996, Gambetta 2007).

Some coaches believe that because the technique between track sprinting and sprinting in field and court sports is different, field and court sport athletes should not be coached on sprinting technique and should just play their sport. This neglects the obvious fact that field and court sports are *running* sports and that speed is a major component of superior performance in a large number of these. To enhance their athletes' performance, coaches should aim to improve their ability to run at speed, or to *sprint*, and to develop this ability within the context of their sport.

Although certain technical variations may exist because of the different demands of track versus field and court sports, several of the fundamental principles of sprinting are common between them. Considering that field and court athletes sprint as part of their sport and that better performers in most

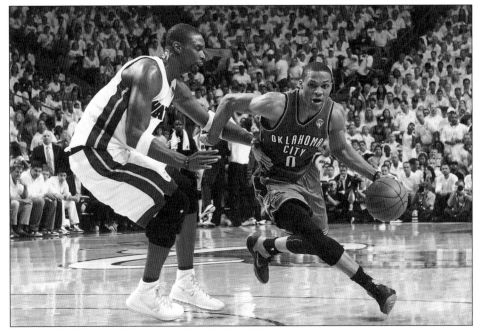

Basketball players like Russell Westbrook use speed and sprinting in combination with other movements, such as cutting, to create lanes to the basket.

field and court sports are faster sprinters (Baker 1999), improving the technical and physical components of sprinting is important within the context of their sport and can give the athletes an advantage over their opponents. Consequently, although many track drills are not suitable for field sport athletes, some common drills and techniques are useful to both the track sprint coach and the strength and conditioning coach working with field and court athletes.

Noted performance enhancement coach Vern Gambetta suggests that the primary coaching points to consider in sprinting are posture, arm action, and leg action (2007). These three considerations are the foundation of effective technique and are discussed in reference to the distinct characteristics of the athlete's posture and arm and leg action in the phases of acceleration, maximal-speed running, and deceleration. In coaching terms, the action of sprinting can also be discussed in terms of back-side and front-side mechanics. Back-side mechanics are the actions occurring behind the body, and front-side mechanics occur in front of the body. Each has different aims, and coaches should focus on the key aims of each.

MAXIMUM SPEED IN FIELD AND COURT SPORTS

Coaches of field and court sports must determine how important the development of maximum speed is. A common perception is that because most maximum sprints in field and court sports are relatively short, maximum speed is relatively unimportant. However, this viewpoint neglects several issues that make the development of maximum speed important to the majority of athletes.

First, elite sprinters achieve very high maximum speeds; therefore, it takes a longer distance for them to reach maximum speed. In the case of male sprinters, this may not occur until 50 to 60 meters. This can be misleading on a number of fronts.

- ▶ Because elite sprinters are faster, they accelerate farther into the race before decelerating; whereas, field and court athletes reach their top speed much sooner, perhaps at 30 to 45 meters.

- ▶ Regardless of whether athletes reach their greatest maximum speed as late as 60 meters or as early as 30 meters into a sprint, athletes are likely running within 10 percent of their maximum speed for half the distance already covered. Therefore, in a 30-meter effort, 15 meters are covered at near maximum velocity.

- ▶ Many sprint efforts in field sports are not initiated from a stationary start. Therefore, when athletes initiate the sprint effort from a jogging or running start, the time and distance needed to reach maximum running velocity is greatly reduced, and so they may run at maximal speeds more often than the recorded distances would suggest.

Second, athletes with higher maximum speeds tend to have a higher rate of change in velocity, which is acceleration. Put simply, the athlete with the highest maximum speed accelerates faster; thereby, sprinting faster at 10 or 20 meters than an athlete with a lower maximum speed.

Finally, higher maximum speed can allow for more effective speed endurance levels during competitions. This is because the relative sprint demands of a field sport are lower for athletes with greater maximum speed because they may not be required to run as many efforts at or even near their own maximum speed. For example, if a rugby player has a maximum speed of 9 meters per second and typically reaches a speed approximately 9 meters per second four to eight times during a game, this presents as a significant stressor. However, if the athlete has a maximum speed of 10 meters per second, efforts involving 9 meters per second are much less stressful because this represents only 90 percent of that athlete's maximum running speed (compared with multiple efforts at 100 percent).

TECHNICAL CONSIDERATIONS FOR SPRINTING PHASES

Proper technique, based on an understanding of mechanical principles, is vital to maximizing running speed. Therefore, developing effective technique is key

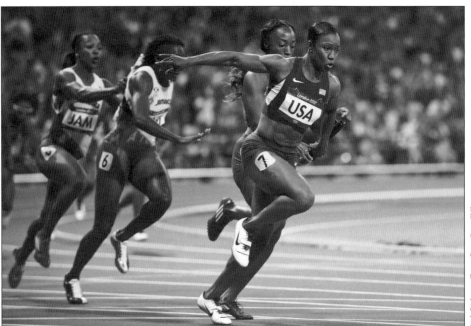

Rick Rickman/Zuma Press/Icon SMI

Even though court and field sports require movements outside of the track sprint, athletes from many sports can benefit from the excellent sprinting techniques that the U.S. Women's relay team displayed at the 2012 Summer Olympics in London.

to any speed enhancement program, and developing technical models of performance should form the basis of training and coaching. Figure 2.1 summarizes the key technical cues for each phase of sprinting, and the exercises outlined in chapter 3 develop the key technical skills of each phase.

For the purposes of this chapter on technical models in accelerating to and running at maximum speed, the emphasis is on the techniques that are effective for straight sprinting (running as fast as possible). Adaptations to these technical models may need to be considered for sports that have specific demands such as carrying a stick or ball, surface conditions, changes of direction, and so on.

Figure 2.1   Key Technical Cues for the Phases of Sprinting

ACCELERATION

- In front of the body, the arms drive forward and upward from the shoulder, in synchronicity with the forward drive of the opposite knee.
- Behind the body the arms drive downward and backward.
- The magnitude of the lean of the body is greatest during initial acceleration, and with each stride the forward lean reduces as the athlete increases running speed.
- The emphasis during acceleration is on back-side mechanics and the pushing action, which is backward and downward. As an athlete accelerates to higher speeds, there is a gradual transition in technique from the form that characterizes early acceleration (pronounced forward lean of the torso; a pushing action of the triple extension of the hip, knee, and ankle behind the body; forward and upward arm action providing propulsion) to that of maximum speed.
- Each stride becomes longer, with less time on the ground as the athlete accelerates. The hips rise with the less acute torso angle, and there is a higher knee lift relative to the hip, with the foot of the recovering leg gaining height with each stride.

MAXIMUM SPEED

- Running position is tall, with the head high and the torso erect.
- The hands reach the level of the face in the front of the body, driving downward and backward first from the shoulder and then with extension at the elbow to the rearward position behind the body.
- Rotation through relaxed shoulders counters the forward rotation through the hips.
- The ankle of the recovery leg (in the swing phase of the stride) travels forward and above the knee of the support leg (in the stance phase of the stride).
- The knee rises in front of the body so that the thigh is a parallel to the ground.
- One foot strikes the ground in front of the other.
- Foot contact is on the balls of the feet. The ankle fully extends at the toe-off position.

DECELERATION

- The athlete absorbs force, primarily through flexion of the ankle, knee, and hip.
- The athlete uses a slight rearward body lean, returning to an athletic position before any subsequent action.
- The arm action aids in the absorption of force and helps maintain balance and control of the body and prepares for subsequent movement (change of direction, skill execution).

Acceleration

Acceleration, as highlighted in chapter 1, is the rate of change in velocity, or the change of velocity in a given time. The first phase of acceleration involves overcoming the body's inertia in order to get moving, as in Newton's first law of motion. Inertia refers to the propensity of a body to resist changes in motion and is at its highest when a body is stationary. Therefore, initiating motion requires great force and depends on maximal strength.

The importance of maximal strength and power during the start and acceleration phase of a sprint can be understood more clearly by remembering that sprinters develop force to overcome inertia when their feet are on the ground. This requires large movements through the hip, knee, and ankle to extend the leg on the ground. Stronger athletes, who can create more force, are better able to use greater forward lean during acceleration. This enables them to assume an effective line of force and minimize the tendency of the body to rotate from side to side, which helps them apply the forces necessary to complete the pushing action in the acute forward lean.

The magnitude of body lean is greatest during initial acceleration. The lean involves the whole body from the ground and not just from the waist (figure 2.2). The athlete is not bent over. The greater the acceleration, the greater the forward lean. Therefore, after the body overcomes inertia and starts moving, the rate of acceleration decreases along with the body lean, and with each step, the body becomes more upright as speed increases.

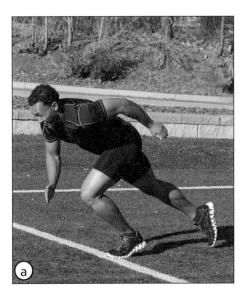 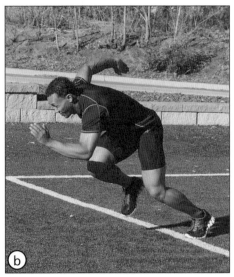

Figure 2.2 Stride sequence from a stationary start, exhibiting forward lean characteristic of acceleration phase.

This gradual transition to a more upright posture and eventually erect running posture coincides with a change in the leg and arm actions from initial acceleration to maximum speed. The hips rise as the torso rises, knee lift is higher relative to the hip, and the foot of the recovering leg (the leg moving forward) gains height with each stride. This transition is a progression to maximum speed technique and doesn't happen all at once. Coaches should not encourage the athlete to stay low. A normal transition to an upright posture takes place and should not be restricted. This is especially pertinent for field athletes who also have to consider the technical requirements of the game and whether staying low will hinder their ability to carry these out.

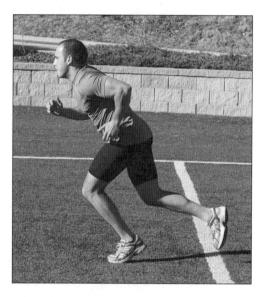

Figure 2.3 Early acceleration stride sequence, exhibiting foot strike with flexed hip and knee.

The first step of a sprint is rapid but relatively short, with a comparatively long ground contact time. Each subsequent step involves a shorter ground contact time and a longer stride length until, ideally, stride length is optimized at maximal speed. During the initial driving strides, the sprinter pushes backward and downward, beginning with a bent knee and flexed hip on contact of the support leg (figure 2.3). The athlete drives the leg back behind the body, fully extending the hip, knee, and ankle to maximize the drive of the legs (figure 2.4). A straight line can be drawn from head to toe running through the hip, knee, and ankle joints.

Fundamental to this technique is having an acute, *positive* shin angle, as illustrated in figure 2.5*a*, when the driving leg contacts the ground.

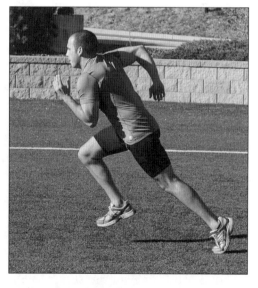

Figure 2.4 Sprinter pushing and extending through hip, knee, and ankle.

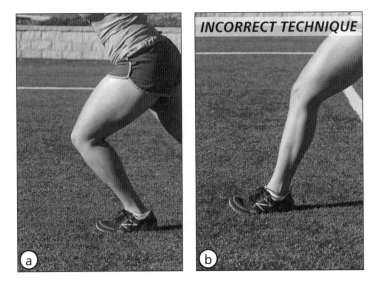

Figure 2.5 Sprinter strides with (a) a positive shin angle that provides the best drive and (b) a negative shin angle that hinders acceleration.

As the athlete accelerates, this angle becomes less acute with each stride to nearly perpendicular at maximum speed. A *negative* shin angle in initial acceleration, as shown in figure 2.5b, indicates that the foot is too far in front of the body to create a pushing action and creates excessive braking forces during foot strike. This means that after the initial foot strike, the athlete has to carry the body over the foot using a relatively weak pulling action before attaining proper posture to apply force backward and downward.

The emphasis of the leg action during acceleration is on back-side mechanics and the pushing action. To achieve this, the arms must propel and lift the athlete during an effective forward lean. Because the force applied to the ground is through the foot, the arm action is sometimes underemphasized. However, the arm drive is fundamental to applying force through the legs, particularly during acceleration, and poor arm action results in inefficient sprint technique.

In front of the body, the arms provide lift when driving forward and upward from the shoulder in synchronicity with the forward drive of the opposite knee (refer to figure 2.4). The arms should remain nearly in line with the shoulders. The rearward drive of the arm downward and backward applies force against the ground, and at this point the athlete opens the elbow angle.

Maximum Speed

Sprint coach Percy Duncan summed up running at maximum speed by saying that "Running occurs *on* the ground. Sprinting occurs *over* it." This statement reflects the concept of an effective sprint position, including posture and arm and leg action, of athletes who have accelerated to near or at their top speed. When a well-trained athlete is running at maximum speed, the body does not oscillate up and down a great deal through the flight phase, hence, the reference to running *over* the ground.

In the strong and well-trained athlete, the body rises through the majority of the flight phase while traveling forward. The athlete's strength and leg stiffness supports the next foot strike with minimal flexion in the ankle, knee, and hip as the foot strike occurs just ahead of the centerline of the body (figure 2.6*a*). The tendency to collapse (excessive flexion of the ankle, knee, and hip) on contact with the ground is characteristic of poorer sprinters and requires a physical development program to supplement the technical program. Figure 2.6*b* illustrates a position in which the foot strike occurs too far ahead of the body, creating large braking (dissipating) forces, increasing ground contact time, and reducing impulse, thereby reducing running speed.

Minimal flexion through the hip and knee during ground contact at maximal speed is a key to elevating the hip. In turn, the elevated hip allows the athlete to drive the leg to nearly full extension (see figure 1.2 in chapter 1). The elevated hip also allows the leg to move freely through an effective range of motion. The ankle of the recovery leg passes above the knee of the support leg (as if stepping over the opposite knee) through flexion at the knee and with the ankle dorsiflexed.

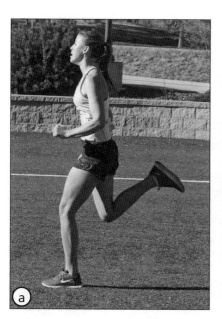
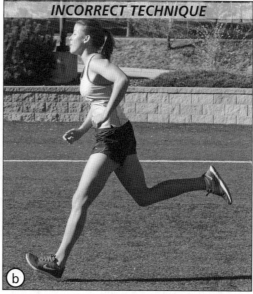

Figure 2.6 *(a)* Correct sprint position with the foot strike just ahead of the body's centerline. *(b)* Poor sprint position with the foot strike too far ahead of the body's centerline.

Flexion of the hip allows the thigh to reach a position parallel to the ground before extension through the hip and ankle as the foot strikes on the ball of the foot just ahead of the body. The high degree of knee flexion in the recovery leg shortens the lever arm, which is critical to producing high stride frequencies.

When running at maximum velocity, the athlete's posture is vertical through the torso, the head is held high, and the shoulders are relaxed. The hands rise in front of the body, level with the chin, driving back first from the shoulder and then with extension at the elbow to a position behind the body.

This motion has been described as the action of a hammer hitting a nail. During maximum speed, the arms come to the centerline of the body through a slight rotation in the shoulder and torso. This rotation counters the rotation of the hips. For this to occur effectively, the shoulders must be relaxed. Raised shoulders restrict their range of motion.

The magnitude of the rotation gradually builds during acceleration; little or no rotation of the hips and shoulders occurs during initial acceleration. The rotation of the shoulders and hips allow the athlete's feet to land nearly one in front of the other (through the rolling of the hip movement), which creates optimal stride length. Restricting this movement through the hips decreases the athlete's stride length and the power from each foot strike, thereby reducing speed.

Deceleration

Deceleration in court and field sports is important when executing certain skills (e.g., a receiver rapidly decelerating to create space from a defender to receive a pass) and to change direction. Depending on the sport, these changes in direction can occur from different approaches. For example, a ball carrier in rugby may decelerate to prepare for a cutting action ahead of a defender, and a tennis player may decelerate and execute a stroke while running laterally.

To decelerate effectively, the athlete must absorb force, primarily through flexion of the ankle, knee, and hip. This action is aided by an initial rearward body lean, which is opposite to that of acceleration. The extent of the lean depends on the initial velocity of the athlete. The muscles in this action decelerate the movement of the body's mass under a high eccentric (lengthening action) load, controlling the rate of deceleration to either a standstill or to a speed at which a change of direction or skill can be executed.

The arms continue to oppose the movements of the lower body, aiding in the absorption of force and providing help to control the athlete's balance and center of mass. Figure 2.7 illustrates the slight rearward lean and flexion (absorption of force) through the lower body to decelerate. Although the initial body lean is rearward, as athletes slow, they are often required to undertake a sport-based task, which requires them to assume a traditional athletic position and the associated forward lean.

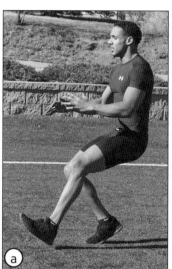
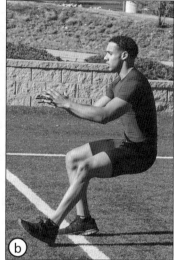
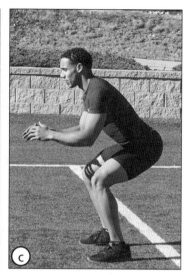

Figure 2.7 Athlete in the *(a)* initial rearward lean, *(b)* transitioning back to the athletic position, and *(c)* in a postdeceleration athletic position.

Common to most situations in which deceleration occurs is the need to initiate a propulsive force soon after the deceleration. For example, an athlete may decelerate and then push off to change direction. Simply put, the athlete must reduce force (decelerate) and produce force (accelerate) in some manner, such as changing direction, jumping, tackling, and so on. Performing this task effectively is a key to multidirectional speed and agility.

The key to reduction and then production of force, as in decelerating from a sprint before changing direction, is using the stretch load inherent to the eccentric action. If used well, the stretch load provided by the eccentric action can contribute greatly to the production of force in the following concentric (shortening) action. Termed a stretch-shortening cycle (SSC), this can greatly enhance force production. SSC function is influenced by the rate, magnitude, and load of the stretch, and depends on a short delay between the eccentric and concentric action. Well-developed technique allows the athlete to decelerate and change direction (or execute another skill) in a superior manner.

When decelerating and absorbing force through the lower body, the athlete must use a range of motion that allows enough lengthening of the muscle to reduce force and stimulate the SSC because the SSC is influenced by the magnitude of stretch. However, too much flexion reduces the athletes' ability to exert concentric force, thereby negating the positive effects of the large magnitude of stretch and increases the delay between the eccentric and concentric action (figure 2.8). Thus, the coaching cue to *sit down low* often results in poor body position. The ideal position depends on the specific requirements of the subsequent action and the specific sport.

A simple method to reinforce this concept is to attempt countermovement vertical jumps from several depths. Attempting a vertical jump from a very shallow dip motion, an extremely deep motion, and then finally from a depth that the athlete feels will illicit the greatest height can help develop this concept. In most athletes, the depth that achieves the greatest jump height is an intermediate dip somewhere between very shallow (minimizing muscle length changes and maximizing speed) and extremely deep (maximizing muscle length changes but reducing speed). This depth optimizes the effective contribution of the SSC while initiating the concentric action from a position in which the muscles can produce force.

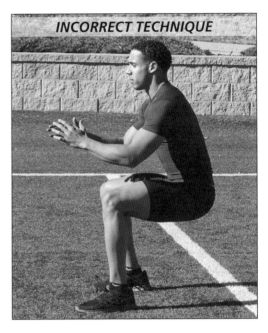

Figure 2.8 Athlete decelerating with extreme flexion through the lower body, reducing the ability to provide enough force to change direction.

The same principle applies to the magnitude of flexion of the ankles, knees, and hips when decelerating. The flexion should be deep enough to dissipate the force through the length of the stretch but not so deep that the body is unable to generate subsequent force effectively.

The physical quality of absorbing, or arresting, force and subsequently accelerating during deceleration and change-of-direction sequences is often referred to as reactive strength. Training this quality includes executing effective technique in decelerating and changing direction. Safely executing this skill requires not only strength in the legs, but also body control and awareness. This is particularly important when considering the importance of reactive agility in many sports, and that during unplanned tasks (reactive changes of direction), the forces that need to be absorbed through the body are much greater than in controlled, planned deceleration, and change-of-direction tasks.

CHAPTER 3

Technical Development of Linear Speed

Jeremy Sheppard

The previous chapters outlined the technical requirements of running speed, and how these are based on fundamental biomechanical principles. This chapter introduces a series of running drills and exercises to develop the technical requirements of effective running speed. It is important to consider at this point that performing running drills does not equate directly to improving running technique. The purpose of a running drill is to emphasize an action or the actions of sprinting as a part of an overall sprint training program. Only when an athlete can perform these correctly and consistently will gains in technical performance be evident.

Along with strength and power training, particular drills assist the coach in advancing sprint technique, but drills should be selected only if the purpose and benefit for the individual athlete is justified. In other words, drills supplement sprint training to achieve specific components of technical and physical development. If a coach cannot justify the use a drill, it's unlikely to be an appropriate drill for that athlete.

Coaches should select drills based on the athlete's needs (particularly technical and physical deficiencies), the sport, and the level of athleticism. As an example, track sprinters' performance is based on running fast, so they need to devote all of their training time to this pursuit in order to maximize these qualities and refine technique to the highest level possible. Therefore, they are likely to perform a large number of technical drills in their training. Field and court athletes have many demands on their training time besides sprint training, so drills for these athletes should focus only on what will provide the largest benefit in technical and physical development. Field and court athletes are likely to perform fewer technical drills than track sprinters because of time limitations (training other skills takes precedence) and their sport-specific fitness needs.

The drills in this chapter are broadly divided into four categories, all with specific goals for speed performance: general, starts and initial acceleration, acceleration to maximum speed, and deceleration. However, in most cases the drills emphasize a particular action that may be common to many aspects of sprinting. The art and science of coaching involves analyzing the deficiencies and needs of an athlete and using the best corrective technique to improve performance.

GENERAL DRILLS

The drills outlined in this section generally serve two purposes: promoting dynamic range of motion and teaching a particular technical aspect. As an example, high-knee drills prepare for the range of motion required for sprinting and teach the knee and arm positions of sprinting, particularly the front-side mechanics. For both track athletes and field and court athletes, these drills are often incorporated into the late stages of the warm-up, before the main speed repetitions of the session. Because the emphasis is on high-quality execution of the drills, coaches should reinforce appropriate technical cues and structure training so that the duration of the repetitions is short to ensure that fatigue does not affect correct technique.

Standing Arm Swing

Aim   This common drill simplifies and isolates the technical cues of the arm swing in sprinting.

Action   The athlete stands in a square or slightly staggered stance and swings the arms back and forth in a relaxed rhythm for 4 to 8 seconds. The hands should come up in front and about even with the chin. The elbows should be bent to about 90 degrees, and the arms should drive from the shoulder and swing rearward from the shoulder back and behind the gluteus, opening somewhat at the elbow on the rearward movement. Some coaches use this drill with light resistance of two to five pounds (1-2 kg) in each hand.

Striding Knee Hug

Aim   This is often used as part of a warm-up before sprinting to develop an effective range of motion during hip flexion.

Action   The athlete stands upright and facing forward. The athlete pulls the knee toward the chest with full hip and knee flexion and fully extends the supporting leg. Upon releasing the leg, the athlete drives it into the ground explosively. The athlete performs the action on the other leg.

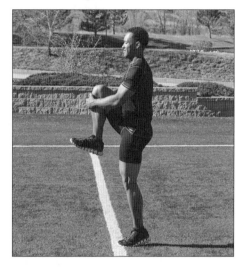

High Knee to Lunge

Aim   To develop effective range of motion, emphasize a tall, high hip position with high knee drive and to emphasize full extension coming out of the deep lunge.

Action   The athlete stands facing forward and drives one knee forward and up, flexing the hip and knee so that the thigh is parallel to the ground and adopting a sprinting arm action (photo *a*). At the same time, the athlete rises onto the toes, emphasizing the extension through the hip, knee, and ankle of the supporting leg. The athlete pauses in the knee-up position, maintaining form while balanced on the balls of the feet, and then drops forward into a deep lunge (photo *b*). The athlete resumes the starting position and repeats on the other side.

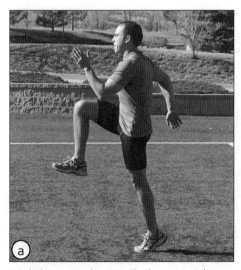

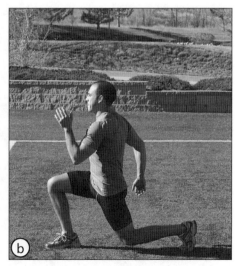

High knee and extended support leg.   Deep lunge.

High Knee

Aim   To develop coordinated front-side mechanics, often used as part of a warm-up and to teach technique.

Action   Several variations of the high-knee drill, including marching As, A skips, and running As are possible. The difference between them is the speed at which they are performed. This drill can be used to learn rhythm and to work on knee lift and leg speed. This is accomplished by performing high knee lifts (marching, skips, or running) at different rhythms. Coaches can choose from several variations. For example, an athlete can perform a high knee drive on only one side or on every second stride on a certain side or alternate from left leg to right leg by performing a high knee every three strides.

Marching As   Marching As use a relatively slow movement emphasizing a high knee lift with full extension of the stance, or supporting, leg. The athlete stands upright facing forward and performs a marching action with each leg. The knee of the lead leg drives up so that the thigh is parallel to the ground (photo *a*). The athlete uses a corresponding arm action, emphasizing full flexion of the arm. When the arm moves to the front, the hand should come up to the chin, and when it moves to the rear, the hand should end behind the hip. On the rear movement, the arm opens slightly at the elbow.

A Skips   The athlete uses the same technique as outlined for marching As, but on each stride, the athlete skips off of the stance leg as the legs alternate, maintaining rhythm throughout the drill (photo *b*). The athlete will achieve a greater degree of extension in the trail leg than in marching As and will leave the ground.

Running As   The athlete uses fast-paced alternation, emphasizing the high knee, fast cadence, and drive downward of the leg. Full extension off of the stance leg lifts the athlete higher in the air than in the previous drills (photo *c*).

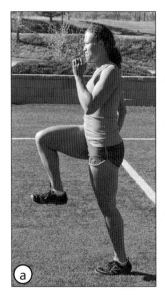 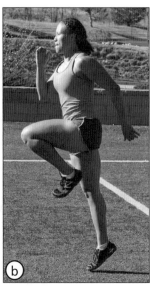 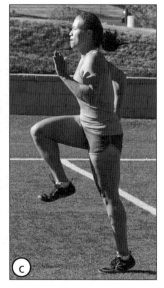

Marching As.   A skips.   Running As.

STARTS AND INITIAL-ACCELERATION DRILLS

As outlined in chapter 1, acceleration is the rate of change in velocity (speed) with respect to time. Whole-body acceleration involves the subtle coordination of the acts of accelerating and decelerating the athlete's limbs to increase the speed at which they move. Although acceleration technique may vary from athlete to athlete because of size and other physical characteristics, there are coachable technical factors that all athletes can develop.

Because acceleration is critical to most sports, understanding and developing acceleration technique is important. One of the primary principles involved in acceleration technique is the forward lean. This forward lean allows the pushing action and other technical considerations outlined in chapter 2. As discussed, during full extension of the leg, a straight line can be drawn from head to foot through the hip and knee (refer to figure 2.4). The stronger and more powerful an athlete, the more forward lean the athlete is able to use, bearing in mind that the greater the rate of acceleration, the greater the forward lean. Therefore, it is important for coaches to increase the strength and power of their athletes, in particular the leg and back muscles, in order to achieve the desired forward lean and full triple extension of the hip, knee, and ankle.

As with any speed session, the importance of high-quality repetitions means that relatively long recovery periods be used between repetitions and sets of drills. When using acceleration-oriented drills that involve running, use distances of 10 to 30 meters. When using explosive drills and those that involve significant sprint movement, perform only a few repetitions in each set. This allows enough rest between sets to maintain high-quality training. A sample session for incline sprints on a five-degree slope would include one or two sets of three or four repetitions of 10 to 30 meters. Rest after each rep would be 3 minutes and rest after each set 5 minutes.

Wall Drive

Aim   To teach or reinforce the posture and leg action in the lean position.

Action   The athlete leans into a wall assuming an acceleration posture, a forward lean with both feet on the ground with weight distributed on the balls of the feet. The athlete alternates bringing the left and right legs forward and up as in a running action. Initially this should be slow and controlled, but as competence increases, the athlete can increase the speed. Athletes who pop up soon after beginning a sprint, thereby using very little forward lean, can benefit greatly from this drill and the associated coaching cues that promote better technique.

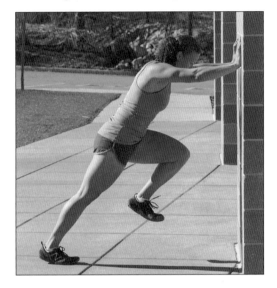

Incline Sprint

Aim   To develop general leg extensor power and to promote the forward lean.

Action   The athlete sprints up a low incline (5-10 degrees), emphasizing effective acceleration action. The added resistance of the incline provides a safe and effective way to stress the strength and power demands of acceleration drills. The upward slope of the surface may also promote an increased awareness of knee drive and full extension while in the forward-lean position. The athlete should walk slowly back to the start to ensure full recovery between efforts.

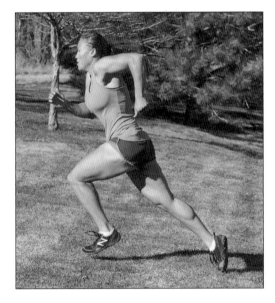

Sprint Starting From the Ground

Aim   To teach effective forward lean in accelerating.

Action   The athlete begins lying facedown on the ground with palms on the ground near the shoulders (photo *a*). On the coach's command, the athlete gets up and sprints as fast as possible to a set point straight ahead (photos *b* and *c*). This distance to the point can vary depending on the aim of the drill, but the distance is normally relatively short, about 5 to 30 meters). Because the athletes begin on the ground, as they raise their body from the facedown position, they will begin striding while the body is low to the ground, pushing back and assuming a forward lean.

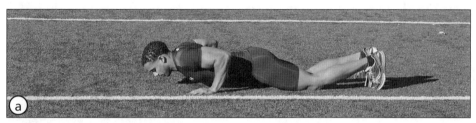

Start position.

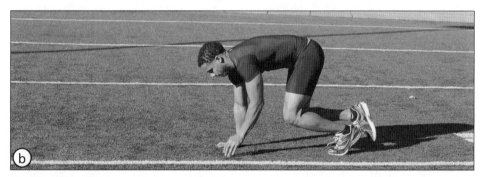

Starting the sprint.

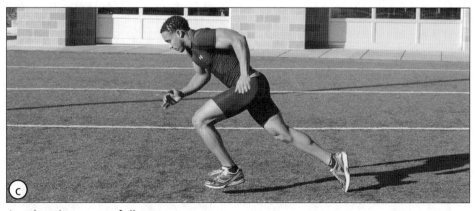

Accelerating powerfully away.

Fall-In Sprint

Aim   To develop acceleration technique, particularly forward lean.

Action   The athlete stands upright and facing forward. Using a whole-body forward lean, the athlete gradually falls forward toward the ground and then accelerates at the last moment for a given distance, such as 10 meters (photos *a* and *b*). A coach or partner can also provide support by holding onto the athlete's shirt to support the forward lean. The coach or partner releases the hold and the athlete accelerates.

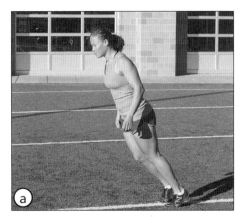
Gradual fall.

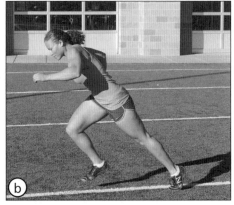
Accelerate powerfully.

Sprint From a Three-Point Start

Aim   To promote the forward lean and the back-side mechanics in acceleration and to emphasize arm drive.

Action   The athlete takes a three-point start position (photo *a*). Driving from this low position, the athlete sprints forward for a given distance, such as 20 meters (photo *b*). (The exact distance depends on whether the athlete needs to work on pure acceleration, transition acceleration, or another phase of sprinting.) Athletes with insufficient arm drive may also benefit from this drill because it promotes propulsion from the arms in order to drive out of the low start position.

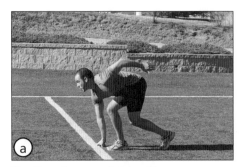
Starting three-point position.

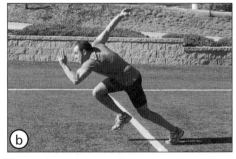
Sprint from low position.

Medicine Ball Squat-Push to Sprint-Out

Aim   To develop the initial explosive action in early acceleration.

Action   The athlete starts in a semicrouched position, holding a medicine ball at the chest with hands placed toward the rear of the ball (photo *a*). The athlete extends fully through the hip, knee, and ankle and extends the arms up, throwing the medicine ball forward, similar to a chest pass, as explosively and as far as possible. On release of the medicine ball, the athlete accelerates 10 to 20 meters (photo *b*).

Medicine Ball Squat-Push to Push-Up Position   The athlete completes the medicine ball squat-push as described, but instead of sprinting after releasing the medicine ball, the athlete drops forward to a push-up position (photo *c*).

Medicine Ball Squat-Push to Dive   This variation requires the use of a high-jump mat placed just in front of the athlete. The athlete completes the drill as described, but instead of sprinting, the athlete finishes the drill by driving the whole body forward explosively and landing on the mat (photo *d*).

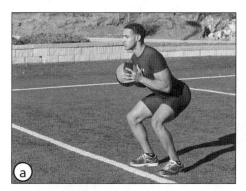

Medicine ball squat-push.

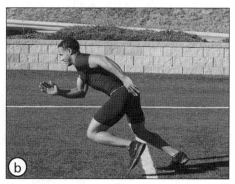

Sprint out.

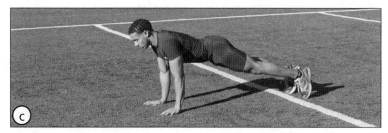

Finish in push-up position.

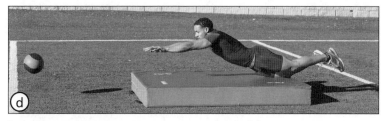

Landing on high-jump mat.

Resisted Sprint

Aim   To develop power for acceleration and to promote appropriate forward lean.

Action   The athlete sprints explosively for a given distance while towing a weighted sled or other similar apparatus. Because of the resistance of the sled, the athlete adopts a slightly exaggerated forward lean. Similar to incline sprints, this is an effective way to develop power and to promote the posture for acceleration. (Greater detail regarding resisted sprints is provided later in this chapter in the resisted sprint section.)

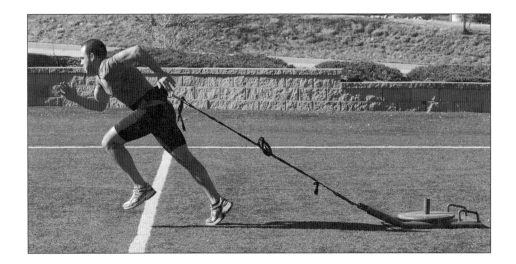

Push Off and Dive

Aim   To develop an explosive push-off action.

Action   This drill is similar to the medicine ball squat-push to dive. The athlete starts in a semicrouched position, drives to an extended position, and then dives onto a high-jump mat (photos *a* and *b*). This drill emphasizes explosive extension at the hip, knee, and ankle, with forward and upward arm drive.

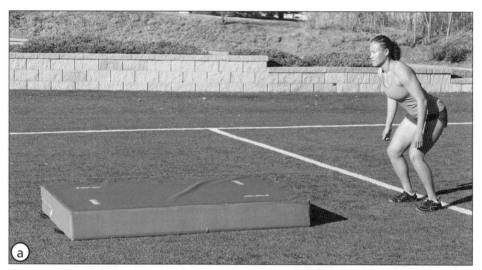

Semicrouched start position.

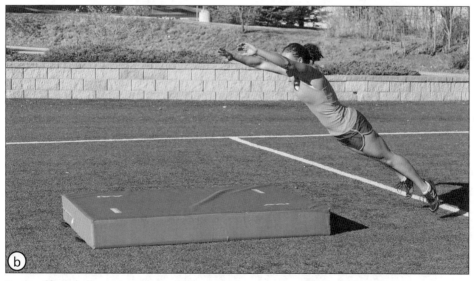

Push off and dive.

Partner Resist-and-Release Start

Aim   To emphasize the forceful drive and pushing actions of acceleration and on release of the resistance to rapidly increase leg speed.

Action   The athlete stands ready to sprint, and the coach stands behind, providing manual resistance by clutching the back of the athlete's shirt or holding onto the hips (photo *a*). The coach provides resistance during the initial acceleration, usually 5 to 10 meters, and then releases the resistance. The athlete continues to accelerate into the sprint for another 10 meters (photo *b*). Another option for providing resistance is a harness. The athlete wears the harness and the coach holds onto a strap attached to it.

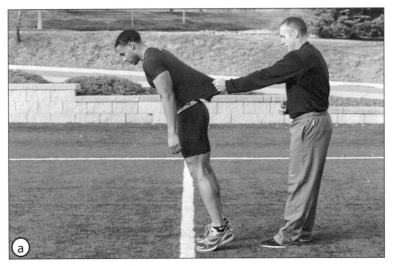

Acceleration under resistance.

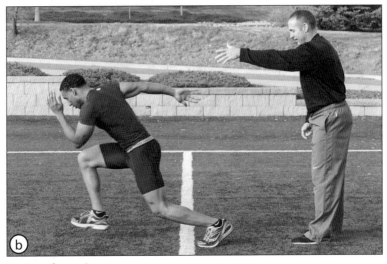

Sprint after release.

ACCELERATION TO MAXIMUM-SPEED DRILLS

Some athletes may be limited in their ability to achieve the technical model outlined in chapter 2 for maximum-speed running because of strength and flexibility limitations. For example, many athletes lack the strength in the hamstrings and flexibility in the quadriceps to flex of the knee of the recovery leg sufficiently to reach maximum speed. Weaker athletes are also unable to provide the propulsion required to optimize stride length (and achieve full extension) and minimize collapsing of the leg on foot strike, resulting in a reduced stride length and excessive up-and-down movement with each stride. Continual evaluation of athletes, recognition of technical limitations and their reason, and then providing training to remedy the limitations are integral components of coaching.

The drills outlined in this section provide a tool for use in a sprint training program. Each activity or drill has a specific purpose, and if appropriate for an individual, may help in supplementing a sprint training program. However, the fundamental component of sprint training is sprinting, so drills should be considered as supplementary.

Sprint Bounding

Aim This action increases leg power and stride length. Because of the ballistic nature of the bounding action, the drill also emphasizes stiffness, particularly at the ankle, during foot strike.

Action The athlete performs an explosive sprint with exaggerated strides for a predetermined distance. For beginners, this distance should be about 10 meters. It can be extended to 30 meters for experienced athletes. The athlete emphasizes a high knee lift and full extension of the drive leg. However, the athlete should not overstride or reach with the forward leg. The stride length is achieved by an emphasis on hopping and very high knee lift. Bounding is a high-intensity exercise and should not be performed unless an athlete has developed effective strength, stretch-shortening cycle ability, and technical capacity for plyometric-based exercises.

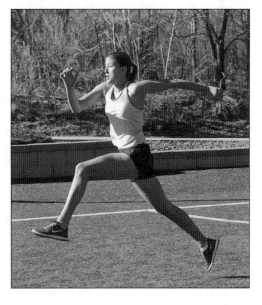

Single-Leg Hop

Aim   To develop leg power while pushing off from the supporting leg and to develop power during the landing and push-off sequence.

Action   The athlete hops on one leg for a given distance, focusing on the height and distance of each hop. During a single-leg hop, the base leg is overloaded, which emphasizes the power in pushing off from that leg. After pushing off, the leg cycles through a motion that includes high knee lift and a high recovery of the ankle after the push-off (photo a). When first learning the exercise, most athletes maintain a low ankle. Before the next foot contact, the athlete brings the ankle up toward the buttocks so it passes higher than the opposite knee and drives the knee of the hopping leg up and forward at the same time. The athlete's foot drives into the ground at a faster and, therefore, more forceful rate than during many other drills because the athlete is actively extending the leg to nearly full extension before landing (photo b). This provides an opportunity to develop the strength and stability of the leg to resist the collapse of the ankle, knee, and hip on foot strike when sprinting and uses the SSC action for propulsion. A useful coaching cue for this drill is to ask athletes to keep their hips high.

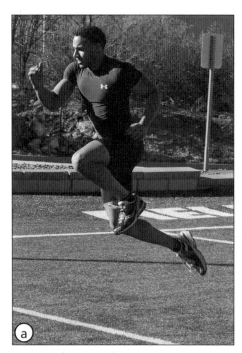

Position for top of hop.

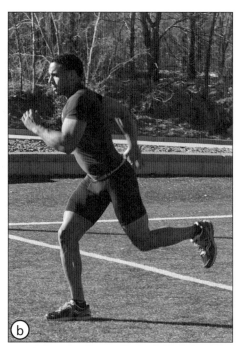

Landing position.

Ankling

Aim To develop elastic strength and general strength in the muscles acting on the ankle.

Action The athlete stands upright then moves forward by alternately flexing and extending the ankle joints. The athlete uses very short steps at a fast cadence, emphasizing brief but explosive contact on the ball of the foot. Throughout the exercise, the hips are high and the knee is nearly extended so that the stress is placed on the muscles acting on the ankle.

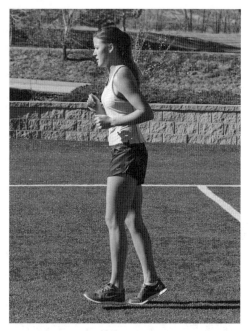

As discussed in chapter 2, not only does acceleration begin from a stationary position (e.g., a track start or a lineman accelerating from the line of scrimmage at the snap) but also from various speeds such as a slow jog (by a rugby forward before ball carry) or a moderate sprint (by a rugby outside back). Acceleration can also follow different movement patterns, such as a receiver running along the line of scrimmage before the snap then turning and sprinting downfield or a rugby forward performing a lateral shuffle away from the ruck to receive the ball and sprint forward.

Performing acceleration drills from specific starting conditions allows evaluation of the athlete's technique for sport-specific situations. In team sports, practicing starts from the relevant start position, in addition to normal skills training, even when athletes may already perform this action in conjunction with skill training, focuses attention on technique and execution. The quality of the athlete's acceleration is affected by the quality of the preceding movement; therefore, a total speed program should address all elements of the athlete's movement. As noted by Gambetta (1996), we must supplement sport training with relevant work on the fundamentals (such as running techniques) in order to advance the athleticism of athletes.

Lateral Shuffle to Forward Sprint

Aim To develop the ability to transition from lateral movement to a forward sprint, a movement required in many sports, particularly American football, rugby, Australian rules football, and similar sports.

Action The athlete shuffles laterally for 5 to 10 meters and then sprint forward for 10 to 20 meters (photos *a* and *b*). Athletes maintain an athletic position while shuffling, with feet facing forward and arms held relaxed in the position of choice for the given sport. Athletes can initiate the forward sprint at a predetermined location or when they have developed effective technique. Athletes can also initiate the forward sprint in reaction to a stimulus.

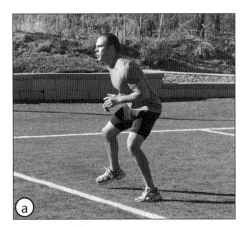
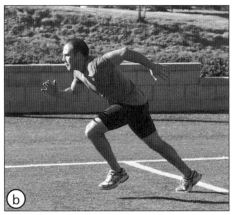

Lateral shuffle.   Sprint forward.

Walk-and-Jog Start to Sprint-Out
(Pick-Up Sprint)

Aim To develop the ability to accelerate from a linear rolling start.

Action Set up two cones about 10 to 20 meters apart. The athlete starts at the first cone and begins walking, eases into a jog, and then shifts to a sprint before reaching the other cone. The athlete focuses on the changes in mechanics associated with changing pace. (Instead of using cones, the coach could cue the transition with relevant commands.)

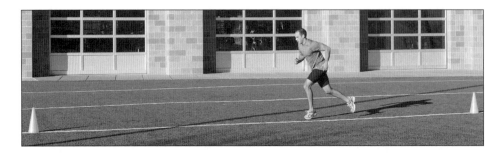

Ins and Outs

Aim   To develop the ability to relax at speed.

Action   The athlete accelerates maximally over 20 meters and then maintains that pace for 20 meters, focusing on relaxing rather than on driving. At 40 meters the athlete accelerates again, trying to reach near top speed as soon as possible after the 40-meter mark and maintains that pace to the 60 meter mark. Finally, the athlete reduces intensity and floats for 10 to 20 meters more, keeping the stride cadence high while focusing on relaxation. The second acceleration gives athletes the opportunity to focus on acceleration mechanics from a relatively fast lead-in speed, improving their transition from a fast run to sprinting and teaching rhythm. The distances of each phase can vary depending on the requirements of the sport and the athlete.

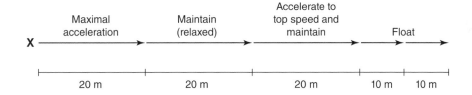

Wall Slide

Aim   To develop a rapid leg recovery.

Action   This drill, which is a variation of the ubiquitous butt-kicker drill, can be carried out while walking, skipping, or running. The major difference is that the athlete does not extend the heels behind the body. Instead, the athlete performs a normal running (or walking or skipping) action but rapidly pulls the heel to the buttock as the knee drives forward. The heel does not extend behind the body, and the ankle is dorsiflexed throughout the movement. Helpful imagery for this drill is a wall at the athlete's back. Each foot slides up the imaginary wall and cannot extend behind the body.

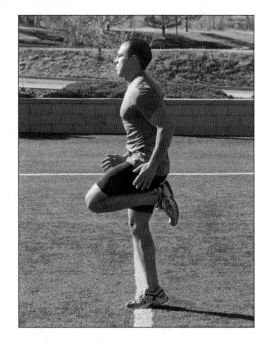

Step Over

Aim To develop a rapid cycling action of the recovery leg.

Action This drill is an extension of the wall slide drill. The athlete performs a normal running action, driving the knee forward and rapidly pulling the heel to the buttock as in the previous drill. Again, the heel does not extend behind the body. In this drill, as the foot comes forward, the athlete extends it out and down as if stepping over something the same height as the opposite knee. The athlete brings the foot down rapidly to make contact with the ground under or just in front of the center of gravity. This drill can be performed statically, walking or running.

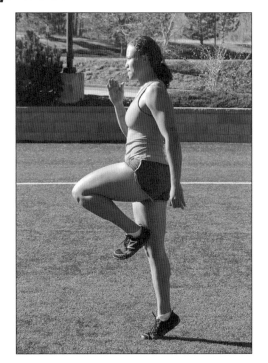

DECELERATION DRILLS

Sprint, deceleration, and change-of-direction drills are popular in training with a sport-specific focus. However, first developing primary strength qualities such as maximal relative strength and reactive strength should not be set aside in an attempt to be sport specific. Doing so could be equated to building the second story of a house before finishing the first floor. Performing endless hours of training for specific applications to their sport is wasted on, and could even be injurious to, athletes who have not developed their foundational strength qualities.

Deceleration in court and field sports allows athletes to change direction and also is critical for executing many sport skills. Depending on the sport, these directional changes can occur from different approaches; therefore, many sport-relevant drills are likely an inherent part of normal training. However, performing drills that emphasize the fundamental technical components outlined in chapter 2 will develop effective technique in the sport-specific application. The drills outlined here are general in sporting application, but are specific to developing deceleration strength and technique. The first three drills (drop landing, drop landing and jump, and drop landing and cut) create a progression.

These deceleration drills are limited to developing fundamental physical and technical components. They do not develop decision-making skills or physical skills in conjunction with a sport-specific perceptual stimulus such as reacting to a ball or an opponent. These should be incorporated into skill training for the athlete's sport. Fundamental movement skills should be seen as a progression from basic abilities fundamental to a skill, to movement patterns broken into components, then through the actual movement at relevant speed and with reaction (Gambetta 2007). The integration of the perceptual and decision-making factors relevant to specific sports is beyond the scope of this chapter.

In addition to the drills provided here, several multidirectional sequences can be used to develop deceleration and change of direction in running. Many common drills exist, including the T drill, L drill, Illinois agility, and proagility. These are useful closed-skill drills that can help develop the fundamental technique of decelerating, changing direction, and accelerating again. These drills can then progress to open-skill deceleration and change-of-direction drills that involve decision making and reaction to a relevant stimulus. The National Strength and Conditioning Association's *Developing Agility and Quickness* is a good resource for learning more about these drills.

Drop Landing

Aim To emphasize the reactive strength involved in arresting movement.

Action The drill is the first step in the drop landing drills and provides practice landing after stepping off a box and stopping the downward movement. The athlete stands on a box 8 to 12 inches (20-30 cm) high. Stronger, well-trained athletes can use boxes up to double that height. Boxes 8 to 24 inches (about 20-60 cm) high in 4-inch (about 10 cm) increments are helpful for monitoring the progression of intensity. The athlete drops from the box and lands on both feet at the same time, absorbing force through the whole body but particularly by flexing the ankles, knees, and hips (photos *a* and *b*). Consider the absorption as optimizing rather than minimizing or maximizing the depth of the squat used to absorb the landing. The athlete uses the arms for balance and progresses from a low height to a higher height. Next, the athlete can progress to single-leg landings, starting with the original lower height (photo *c*).

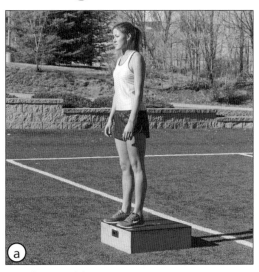
a

Starting position.

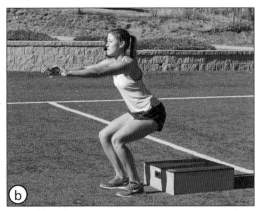
b

Regular drop landing.

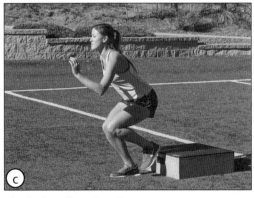
c

Single-leg drop landing

Drop Landing and Jump (Depth Jump)

Aim To emphasize the reactive strength involved in arresting movement.

Action This drill uses the drop landing drill setup and technique. For this progression, the athlete drops from the box and on landing, uses the stretch load provided by the drop to enhance the SSC function and to produce an explosive jump. The athlete should land and jump fluidly, jumping as high as possible. This type of training increases reactive strength for tasks requiring a run–decelerate–jump sequence (Sheppard et al. 2008a, Sheppard et al. 2008b).

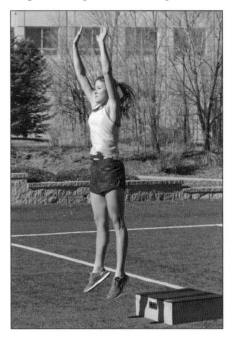

Drop Landing and Cut

Aim To emphasize the reactive strength involved in arresting movement and initiating a cut.

Action The final progression adds a cutting action to the sequence. The athlete drops and lands on both feet (as in the drop landing), then cuts to the right or left, driving off of the opposite foot and stepping out with the foot that is in the direction of the movement (photo *a*). A more advanced version uses a single-leg landing from a relatively low height (20 cm) and cuts to the opposite direction (photo *b*).

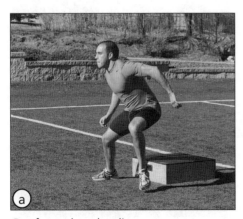

Cut from drop landing.

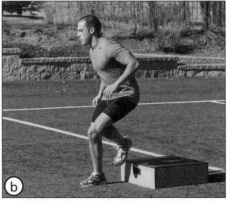

Cut from single-leg drop landing.

Forward–Backward Acceleration and Deceleration

Aim To isolate simple acceleration and deceleration mechanics when running forward and backward.

Action Set up eight cones in a straight line 5 to 10 feet (2-3 m) apart, numbering them 1 to 8 down the line. The athlete starts next to the line of cones, between cones 4 and 5 and facing cone 8. The athlete sprints forward to cone 5 (the closest cone), decelerates and then backpedals to cone 4. The athlete decelerates and then sprints forward to cone 6 and then backpedals to cone 3. The athlete continues this pattern, sprinting forward to cone 7, backpedaling to cone 2, sprinting forward to cone 8 and back pedaling to cone 1. In this manner, the athlete sprints forward and backward from short to longer distances. The drill can also be performed in the opposite sequence, longer to shorter distances. The total sequence constitutes one repetition, which can be repeated for the required number of repetitions.

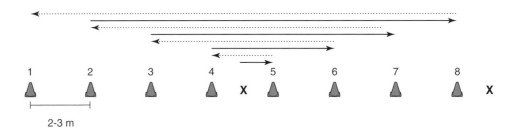

Lateral Acceleration and Deceleration

Aim To develop lateral acceleration and deceleration mechanics.

Action The sequence described in the forward–backward acceleration and deceleration drill can also be performed using lateral movement. Some sports, such as ice hockey, may indicate that a crossover step (see photo) be used. Athletes from other sports should use a standard side shuffle (e.g., rugby players).

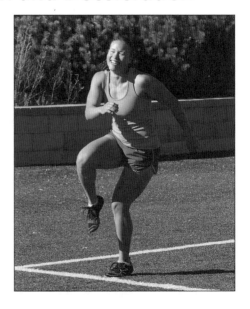

Lateral Stepping

Aim To develop the ability to move laterally in an explosive manner.

Action The athlete bounces from left leg to right leg, jumping laterally and aiming to increase height and distance. The athlete begins slowly in order to master the technical concept and then progresses to a ballistic action back and forth, increasing the height and distance of each jump with the speed of each step.

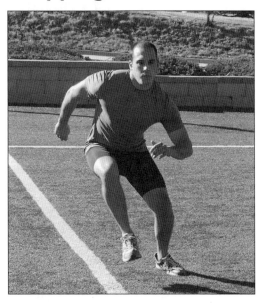

Zigzag Bound (Outside Bounding)

Aim To develop reactive strength in a manner similar to a deceleration and change-of-direction sequence.

Action The athlete runs 5 meters and then bounds at an angle (the zig) by bouncing from one leg to the other, jumping as far as possible. On foot contact, the athlete immediately bounds to the opposite side (the zag pattern), landing on the opposite foot. The foot-strike pattern is outside of the normal position to introduce a slight lateral component into the bounding exercise. The athlete should aim to bound for as great a distance as possible while maintaining control of the landing.

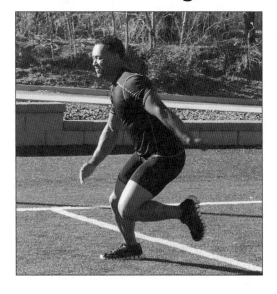

DESIGNING SPEED TRAINING SESSIONS

The greatest gains in sprint performance come from high-quality training characterized by a technical focus, high-intensity efforts, and long recovery periods. Another way to measure quality in sprinting is by how fast an athlete runs. In simple terms, poor speed is poor quality, so everything possible must be done to maximize sprint quality during sessions.

Maximizing sprint quality requires carefully planning of training volume not only for each session but also for longer training periods. If the weekly or monthly sprint volume is too great, the first sprint effort of a new session will be of poor quality because the athlete was unable to recover between sessions, and this may also increase the risk of injury. Tolerance of training volume is highly individual and is influenced by training history and genetic factors. However, generally speaking, 1,000 to 2,000 meters per week of acceleration and high-speed sprinting is typical.

Tables 3.1 and 3.2 outline two sample sprint sessions, including warm-up and drill sequences. Both sessions include common elements, but table 3.2 demonstrates the negative effect that inadequate rest can have on the athlete, despite the fact that the sessions are relatively low in total sprint volume.

One of the most important principles to understand when designing speed training sessions is the impact of high-intensity effort on an athlete. Sprint training applies a large stressor to the central nervous system and peripheral nervous system. Coaches may overlook or underestimate this because the total work (duration of effort or distance covered) is relatively small compared to other types of training. It is helpful to remember that the classic super-compensation curve is a theoretical model and that, in fact, each type of training stress elicits a different compensatory response. For example, most athletes can perform a nonsprinting running session and recover enough to repeat or exceed the intensity within 24 hours. However, evidence has shown that a typical sprint session, where intensities are 95 to 100 percent, often requires rest from sprinting for 72 hours or more and certainly not less than 48 hours. Elite sprinters who have performed at a personal-best level may need as much as 10 days of rest from sprinting. The ability to recover from a high-intensity sprint session is also determined by the volume of work carried out, which influences the total stress. For example, a high-intensity (95-100% of max speed) session of 300 meters requires less recovery time than a 750-meter session similar in nature.

Table 3.1 Low-Volume, High-Quality Sprint Session

Activity	Volume	Rest	Time (sec.)
WARM-UP			
Slow jog	800 m		
Static stretch	10 min.		
Dynamic stretch	10 min.		
Hurdle walk-over	2 × 10 m	1 min.	
A skip	3 × 20 m	1 min.	
Medicine ball squat-push	3 × 10	30 sec.	
Sprint bounding	3 × 30 m	2 min.	
ACCELERATION			
Sprint from a 3-point start	20 m	3 min.	3.08
Sprint from a 3-point start	20 m	3 min.	3.04
Sprint from a 3-point start	20 m	3 min.	3.05
5-minute rest			
STARTS			
Blocks	30 m	5 min.	4.44
Blocks	30 m	5 min.	4.42
Blocks	30 m	5 min.	4.41
10-minute rest			
FLYING EFFORTS			
30-meter build up	20 m	7 min.	2.24
30-meter build up	30 m	10 min.	3.39
30-meter build up	40 m		4.65

Table 3.2 High-Volume, Low-Quality Sprint Session

Activity	Volume	Rest	Time (sec)
WARM-UP			
Slow jog	800 m		
Static stretch	10 min.		
Dynamic stretch	10 min.		
Hurdle walk-over	2 × 10 m	1 min.	
A skip	3 × 20 m	1 min.	
Medicine ball squat-push	3 × 10	30 sec.	
Sprint bounding	3 × 30 m	2 min.	
ACCELERATION			
Sprint from a 3-point start	20 m	2 min.	3.07
Sprint from a 3-point start	20 m	2 min.	3.08
Sprint from a 3-point start	20 m	2 min.	3.10
3-minute rest			
STARTS			
Blocks	30 m	3 min.	4.48
Blocks	50 m	3 min.	4.47
Blocks	30 m	3 min.	4.50
5-minute rest			
FLYING EFFORTS			
30-meter build up	20 m	4 min.	2.27
30-meter build up	30 m	4 min.	3.42
30-meter build up	40 m		4.68

SPEED ENDURANCE

Most athletes require some form of speed endurance. Speed endurance can be looked at in two ways: the ability to maintain speed over a single sprint bout (eg a 20 metre sprint) or the ability to maintain speed over repeated shorter bouts as required in many sports such as American football. In track, the level of speed endurance required depends on the sprint event: the 400 meters requires more speed endurance than the 200 meters, and the 200 meters more than the 100 meters. Because speed endurance training is a high-intensity effort, it is considered speed work and not an endurance-oriented endeavor in which volume is the primary outcome. It is imperative to apply the principle of high-quality training to speed endurance sessions. (For more information about designing endurance training programs, see *Developing Endurance* by the NSCA.)

It is common practice to precede speed endurance sessions with general sprint technique drills and starts. However, simply adding speed endurance efforts to the end of speed sessions is not likely to produce favorable results. Consider these two speed endurance workout options:

Session 1: 5 × 120 meters at approximately 95 percent of best time with 7 to 10 minutes rest between sets

Session 2: 2 × 300 meters at approximately 95 percent of best time with 10 minutes rest between sets

Both are typical sessions that could be carried out at the end of a speed training session. If either session, both totaling 600 meters, were added to a typical 600- to 900-meter sprint session of acceleration and top-speed sprinting, the time targets for the speed endurance repetitions would likely be unattainable, due to the overall volume of sprint work required. In addition, many coaches, including the author, have found out how easy it is to tear an athlete's hamstring conducting sessions this way.

It could be said that if sprinters have three gears, they should only use first gear, less than 70 percent of top speed (a low-intensity tempo session), for recovery and general conditioning and use third gear, more than 95 percent of top speed, for speed development. Second gear, or moderately intense running, is too slow to improve an athlete's speed, but challenging enough to present a considerable metabolic and neuromuscular stress. Speed endurance is also influenced by how fast the athlete is. The faster the athlete, the longer he or she accelerates and the later he or she reaches maximal speed; therefore, speed endurance is not a component of the event for as long. Considering this, using moderately intense running to develop speed endurance does not make sense. Because the running is too slow, the training results in an ability to endure slowness.

DISTRIBUTION OF SPEED WORK

How speed work is distributed through the week depends on how many sessions of high-intensity work will take place. Typically, two or three speed sessions are conducted per week when the primary focus is on speed development. Whether to conduct two or three depends on the recovery and performance capabilities of the athlete. Athletes should perform speed sessions on nonconsecutive days, the allocation depending on the number of sessions to be performed and the distribution of other conditioning and skill-based training.

When two sessions take place, it is relatively easy to ensure adequate recovery between the two high-intensity days by scheduling strength training instead of running sessions later in the same day of both of the speed sessions. Tempo runs can take place on consecutive days, and conditioning exercises, such as abdominal work and low-intensity drills that have a low stress on the central nervous system, can also be implemented. Depending on the athlete's training priorities, both speed sessions can emphasize acceleration and speed, or one session can emphasize acceleration and speed and the second session emphasize starts and speed endurance.

RESISTED SPRINTS

Resisted training applies an external resistance to a natural sprint performance. External resistance can be achieved through a variety of methods, such as running uphill, running with a parachute, or towing an external load in the form of a sled. This section focuses on the latter because it has been the focus of the most research. Resisted sprint training methods have been addressed in coaching literature, and there is concern that these methods can result in biomechanical changes in technique. Several studies have outlined the biomechanical changes that take place under resistive conditioning in sprinting.

Research suggests that the changes in the biomechanics during resisted sprints (increased knee flexion at foot strike and increased forward lean) are proportional to the load used and can increase ground contact time. In light of this and coaching observations, it has been suggested that resisted methods only be used with mature athletes who have established a foundation in sprinting and who are, therefore, less likely to be negatively influenced by the biomechanical variations that this type of training imposes.

Indeed, an entirely justified emphasis is placed on developing the biomotor abilities during the formative years, especially sprinting technique. Attempting to overload athletes in a manner that alters their technique before they have developed near optimal form is not recommended. However, with a fully developed athlete, whose movement patterns in the sprint are already highly developed, it is less likely that a conservative volume and load of resisted or assisted sprinting would alter his or her technique under normal sprint conditions.

Coaches develop the qualities required for a specific sport by creating a challenge (overload) and using methods that are specific to the sport. Overload and specificity are the premises behind training techniques such as resisted sprinting; they impose an overload in a manner that is specific to sprinting. When using resisted sprint training, such as towing a weighted sled, the extra load demands that the athlete produces greater force.

A load that is too great, though, imposes biomechanical changes on sprint technique, and it is not known whether this alteration negatively affects technique in the long term. Therefore, resisted sprints should be performed with relatively low loads. A common suggestion is a load of up to 10 percent of body mass.

Most coaches who use resisted sprints use them to develop the initial start and early acceleration phase of sprinting. This practice is supported by studies that demonstrate that the positive benefits of resisted sprinting are associated with improved start and acceleration times over the first 30 meters of a sprint. However, other studies, have shown no improvement in high-speed sprinting with resistance, and so it is still difficult to provide conclusive evidence of the benefit of resisted training in a speed training program.

Coaches and athletes should be aware that the method used to provide resistance affects the load imposed on the athlete. When using rubber resistance bands, the resistance increases as the athlete accelerates away from the fixed end of the band, so the relative feel of the resistance is closer to constant. When using a sled, the relative load is highest at the start and during initial acceleration because of the need to overcome inertia. Another consideration when using a sled is the friction created between the ground and the sled. For example, a smooth wooden sled on certain synthetic surfaces creates less friction than the same sled on a running track. Coaches should consider these influences on the relative load imposed. They could monitor these factors by examining the decrease in sprint time when using resistance compared to normal. A load that reduces sprint time by 1 to 10 percent is a relatively low-resisted sprint load.

A dearth of training studies compare the effects of low- and high load resisted sprinting. Although it is understood that resisted sprint loads greater than 20 percent of body mass elicit significant changes in sprint technique (Maulder et al. 2008 and Knicker 1994), it is not known whether the heavy loads produce a favorable training effect or whether the negative effects on technique outweigh the potential benefits. It is possible that heavy resistance loads, although altering technique during the resisted effort, provide a positive training effect and do not create long-term unfavorable changes in sprint technique. It can also be argued that resisted methods such as towing a sled and sprinting up an incline teach awareness of technical cues for acceleration: pronounced forward lean, full extension of the leg in the stance phase, and a pronounced hip drive. If used sparingly, sprints using heavy resistance can develop certain technical aspects of sprint technique without long-term negative effects. However, little evidence exists to support the use of heavy resistance in sprint training.

ASSISTED SPRINTING

In assisted sprinting, external forces enable the athlete to achieve supramaximal speeds. The goal of the assistance is to enhance speed by increasing stride frequency and is generally provided by towing the athlete by a piece of rubber tubing or by running on a slight decline. However, the benefit of this training method is not well understood. Assisted sprints decrease ground contact time and increase flight time and stride length. Concern exists that some assisted sprinting methods, particularly downhill sprinting, encourage overstriding, which is detrimental to developing the sprint mechanics that produce top speed. During downhill sprints the athlete reaches with the foot to make contact with the ground that is relatively far away from their body because of the slope. This results in a foot strike farther ahead of the center of gravity than in normal high-speed sprinting.

Because of the lack of clear benefits and the limitations of assisted sprinting, some coaches do not recommend it and enhance stride frequency through directed drills that allow for greater than normal rates in specific components of the sprint cycle (Francis 1997). Indeed, many drills that use just a portion of the entire range of motion of a sprint stride allow an increased rate of leg turnover. As with other specialized training methods, assisted sprinting should only be used for highly competent athletes with well-developed technique.

Another method of assisted sprinting free of the pitfalls that may be associated with downhill sprinting, is wind assistance. Athletes run faster with a tailwind, possibly because of reduced ground contact time and increased stride length. A tailwind applies the assistance to the whole body and not a particular point of stress, which may prevent or minimize negative alterations to sprint technique. However, this is extremely difficult to apply in a training context since you cannot plan for the wind conditions.

CHAPTER 4

Assessment of Speed

John Graham

An important element of designing training programs to enhance speed is the ability to assess an athlete's speed and performance levels so that appropriate training decisions can be made. Assessment administrators with an understanding of exercise physiology can use the results of sport performance assessments to make training decisions that will help their athletes to achieve performance goals and maximize potential (Graham 1994, Harman 2008). Results of sport performance assessments form the foundation for training programs and also provide an objective means of determining the success of a training method.

RATIONALE

An assessment is simply a way to measure one's ability in a particular endeavor, in this case athletic performance. Effective assessment brings a number of advantages, and coaches can use speed assessments for a range of reasons, such as evaluating athletic ability, aiding in motivation, and identifying strengths and weaknesses of their athletes (Graham 1994, Harman 2008). Performance results should serve as a basis for developing individual strength and conditioning programs. Once baseline measurements have been established for each athlete, achievable goals can be set, and future assessments can indicate progress toward reaching those goals.

Assessment can also serve as a motivational tool because it is probably the most effective and accurate means of documenting and measuring progress and, therefore, adherence to the program. Goal-oriented athletes recognize the importance of positive assessment results and tend to be competitive in their desire to achieve the best rating (Bridgman 1991).

Tests can also help coaches organize groups. Based on the results, the coach can determine appropriate training partners and can group athletes of similar abilities together. Assessment results can help coaches match athletes with others that will provide them the greatest training benefit.

Assessments can also predict whether an athlete has the skills or physical potential to play a sport at a competitive level, especially where athletes' test results can be compared against norm scores for a specific sport or playing positions (Harman 2008). Because speed plays an important role in many sports, it is essential for both the sport coach and the assessment administrator to be able to accurately assess an athlete's speed, and this requires them to know how to set up valid and reliable speed assessment protocols.

PREREQUISITES

For a testing regimen to be of use to athletes and coaches, the testing protocol must meet several prerequisites. Assessments must be valid, reliable, and objective in order to produce acceptable measurements for evaluation (Graham 1994, Harman 2008). Unless the issues of validity, reliability, and, where appropriate, objectivity are addressed, testing results will be flawed and, thus, the usefulness of the tests severely compromised.

Validity

Validity refers to the degree to which an assessment measures the characteristic it is intended to measure. Four considerations affect the validity of speed tests:

▶ **Construct validity**—whether the speed test actually measures running speed that relates to performance in a specific sport

▶ **Predictive validity**—how the performance on the speed test relates to performance in the sport itself

▶ **Content validity**—how important the speed test selected is to the specific sport

▶ **Concurrent validity**—whether a relationship exists between the speed test and other accepted methods of assessment.

To better understand the validity of an assessment, consider the use of a 30-yard dash as a speed assessment for baseball players. The 30-yard dash has construct validity because it measures a skill commonly used in baseball: running speed between the bases. An athlete with an excellent score in the 30-yard dash theoretically has an advantage in baseball compared to someone with a lower score, therefore, giving the test predictive validity. A 30-yard dash has content validity because it measures running speed, an important criterion in baseball. Finally, the 30-yard dash measured by electronic timing provides concurrent validity by ensuring that the times recorded are accurate and relate to the times that would be recorded with the gold-standard timing systems used at track meets. However, while the 30-yard dash has clear validity for a baseball player, its validity for a basketball player is not so clear because the typical distances run in basketball are far shorter. For basketball, a 10-yard dash may offer a greater degree of validity.

Reliability

In athletic performance assessment, reliability refers to the degree of consistency in results during repeat assessments. In our example of a 30-yard dash, an athlete performing three 30-yard dashes with an adequate recovery between them should ideally achieve the same score in each trial. In reality, there is always an error score in a test, but a tester should try to minimize the error score by controlling as many of the variables as possible. Scoring deviations or measurement error can include inconsistency in athletic effort, examiner error, instrument malfunction, and calibration error. While some of these are difficult to control (e.g., athlete effort), others are controllable (e.g., test protocols) and need to be considered before setting up a speed assessment. This chapter describes how to construct tests that maximize reliability by addressing the controllable variables, thus producing effective results on which to base evaluation and program design.

Objectivity

Objectivity is the level to which multiple assessors agree on the scoring of tests; in essence, it is a specific type of reliability. To optimize objectivity, wherever possible, one designated assessor should be used. Where repeated tests are required, testing programs should aim to use the same assessor for both initial and follow-up examinations, but this is not always possible. A consistent level of objectivity is critical when more than one assessor is used, and all assessors need to be trained to run all the tests. In these situations, it is best to use a predetermined scoring system, fixed and clear testing protocols, and identical instruments to maximize objectivity. For example, the assessor should know exactly how to set up timing gates, execute the required start protocols, score tests accurately, and so on.

In addition to the issues of objectivity associated with the administration of a test, it is important to address potential issues in score reporting. To avoid inaccurate reporting of assessment results, an unbiased tester should be used wherever possible. It is not uncommon for recorded scores or times to be inaccurately reported for the sake of pleasing a coach or parent. Inflating the scores prevents athletes from understanding their performance and can lead to disappointment in the future. In addition, inaccurate scoring negatively affects national statistical norms if these scores are used to generate this data. This could lead to the perception that the athletes or strength coaches at a particular school, who are conducting assessments correctly, are below par.

SELECTION

When selecting assessments, the assessment administrator should analyze the speed demands of the sport the athlete participates in. For example, while a 40-yard dash provides an excellent field test for measuring speed for an American football skill position, it does not offer the same validity for a softball player, who typically sprints just 20 yards to the next base, including decelerating to a stop.

When choosing speed assessments, assessment administrators should make sure that the tests are not only valid, reliable, and objective but also are simple and interesting and provide a positive experience for the athletes (Howley and Franks 2003). A test should be simple and economical; this will ensure rapid and efficient administration to large groups without the need for expensive or complicated equipment. The assessment should appeal to the competitive instincts of the athletes so that they will apply maximum effort and should provide an experience designed to enhance their physical development.

When selecting assessments, several variables need to be considered:

▶ **Age.** Assessments that are valid for college athletes may not be appropriate for adolescents, who lack experience and perhaps motivation (AAHPERD 1980). An example might be to use a 30-yard dash for high school and college baseball players but only a 20-yard dash for Little League athletes who play on smaller fields.

▶ **Gender.** Some assessments may be appropriate for men but not for women or vice versa. For example, a 30-yard dash would be an appropriate assessment for older baseball players, who run 30 yards between bases, but not for softball players, who run just 20 yards from base to base.

▶ **Experience.** Advanced assessments may prove too difficult for novice athletes, for example, using 20-yard assessments for youth soccer players, who compete on smaller fields, instead of the 40-yard assessments used for high school and college soccer players.

▶ **Environment.** Certain assessments may not be appropriate when experiencing environmental extremes such as high altitude or excessive heat and humidity. For example, assessment administrators should avoid assessments outdoors on excessively cold or hot days or days with rain or snow to prevent injury and to improve test validity. Additionally, wind creates a massive variable in performance. Indoor testing can provide more reliable results than outdoor testing because more variables can be controlled.

▶ **Sport-specific characteristics and positions within a sport.** Different sports require adjustments to the test to reflect typical patterns of speed within that sport. For example, because playing basketball typically requires short accelerations, the best speed assessment would be a short test, such as 10 yards. And baseball speed should be assessed by a longer test: 30 yards to match the distance between bases. Additionally, players of different positions within a sport might require different skills and, therefore, different assessments. For example, coaches might use a 40-yard dash for a skilled position in football, and a 10-yard dash might better assess the speed of linemen.

▶ **Unbiased assessment.** An assessment should be specific to the activity and the energy system the athlete has trained. For example, basketball players never run farther than 90 feet (about 30 meters). As a result, testing the 40-yard-dash speed for basketball players would not be a wise choice.

▶ **Instrumentation.** Differences in running speed are often marginal, so accurate measurement and evaluation are crucial. Although assessment administrators often use stopwatches, the potential for error is large, especially when the tester is untrained. Research has demonstrated that, even with experienced test administrators, times recorded by a handheld stopwatch may be .20 seconds faster than those measured electronically over the same distance. This is probably caused by the test administrators' reaction time when pressing the start and stop button at the beginning and completion of the sprint (Harman 2008, Hoffman 2006). Additionally, handheld stop watches potentially allow for tester bias, where the tester consciously or subconsciously manipulates the score. If possible, electronic timing should be used. Increasingly low-cost options for electronic timing equipment are available and offer far greater accuracy over a stopwatch.

▶ **Test protocols.** Protocol can significantly affect the results of a test. For example, the score on a 30-yard dash preceded by a 5-yard running start differs greatly from a 30-yard dash performed from a three-point start. Therefore, the protocols used for each test must be identical and accurately recorded for every athlete and every time the test is given. Recording the test protocol allows other testers to adhere to the same protocol each time the testing is conducted. Variation in protocol makes it difficult to compare scores between different programs and to generate norms.

FREQUENCY

Determining how often to set up athletic performance assessments is important. The coach must have a clear rationale for testing, and this rationale should guide the testing program. Testing for testing's sake is never justified, and all testing programs should work toward a clear goal.

Many coaches assess their athletes three or four times a year; others assess more or less frequently (Bridgman 1991). Some coaches assess every couple of weeks, and still others test only before the sport season. While three or four times a year is often recommended, this is not a hard-and-fast rule; instead, a testing program should be led by the aims of the training program. Testing also can take place naturally through the training period and does not have to consist of a deliberately set aside protocol. For example, if athletes perform sprint activities as part of their training, coaches can measure some of these if data on performance is required.

Coaches should consider two factors when determining testing frequency. First, if formal testing takes place too frequently, valuable training time is lost, and athletes do not receive the same level of performance enhancement from assessments as they do from training (Bridgman. 1991). Second, when athletes are assessed only before preseason camp, they may be less motivated to perform off-season strength training and conditioning. Also, when testing only before the preseason, program changes that could have been made during the off-season are never made, thus neglecting athletes' weaknesses that need attention.

I recommend assessing athletes three times a year: at the end of the season, at the end of the off-season, and at the end of the preseason (Graham 1994). Testing at these points provides the assessment administrator an opportunity to take advantage of the active-rest phase between periods. This enables an accurate assessment from the training period just completed so that adjustments can be made for the next period and for that same training period in the following year's program. Additionally, for sports that have an extended season, adding an in-season test to assess speed function during the season can reveal adjustments that may be needed.

Performing assessments three times annually motivates athletes to continue training during the season, off-season, and preseason and makes each assessment event particularly important. Ideally, assessments are conducted often enough to accurately measure an athlete's progress and the effectiveness of the strength and conditioning program. Assessments should also sustain the athlete's motivation and adherence to the program.

ORGANIZATION AND PREPARATION

Once the assessments have been chosen, an organized format ensures the proper preparation of facilities, assessment administrators, and athletes. Areas to address include the following:

▶ Pretesting protocols
▶ Facility and equipment preparation
▶ Test administration and documentation
▶ Sequencing
▶ Athlete preparation
▶ Score recording

Pretesting Protocols

To ensure participation, in and to develop enthusiasm for, the assessment process, coaches should announce the assessment date at least three weeks before the assessment, and post information about the test in a highly visible area that participants use frequently. The schedule should include details of the assessment; list athletes to be assessed; the name of the assessment administrator; and the location, date, and time of the assessment. Table 4.1 provides a sample schedule for baseball testing and provides information for both administrators and participants. In some instances, coaches may want to separate the information for participants and administrators into two separate checklists. To maximize the effectiveness of the testing session, especially when athletes are being tested for the first time, coaches and assessment administrators can hold a meeting a few days before the test to demonstrate all the tests, answer questions, and explain guidelines and procedures.

All athletes should sign an informed consent form or have a parent or guardian sign it if they are high school level or younger. The form will identify medical conditions that may lead to injury or hinder performance. Informed consent forms also give young athletes and their parents a description of the procedure. A copy of all test procedures and guidelines and the purpose of the assessments should be attached to the consent form. A checklist for the athletes is also recommended (see figure 4.1).

Table 4.1 Testing Schedule: Baseball

Test	Test administrator	Location	Date and time	Athlete group	Equipment needed
Proagility	Jones	Baseball field	Sat., Sept. 7, 9:00 a.m.	Pitchers, catchers	Clipboards, pencils, worksheets, electronic timers, 3 cones
			Sat., Sept. 7, 9:30 a.m.	Position players	
L drill	Ruiz	Baseball field	Sat., Sept. 7, 9:00 a.m.	Position players	Clipboards, pencils, worksheets, electronic timers, 3 cones
			Sat., Sept. 7, 9:30 a.m.	Pitchers, catchers	
30-yard dash	Thomas	Baseball field	Sat., Sept. 7, 10:00 a.m.	Pitchers, catchers	Clipboards, pencils, worksheets, stopwatch, 4 cones
			Sat., Sept. 7 10:30 a.m.	Position players	
60-yard dash	Johnson	Baseball field	Sat., Sept. 7, 10:00 a.m.	Position players	Clipboards, pencils, worksheets, stopwatch, 4 cones
			Sat., Sept. 7, 10:30 a.m.	Pitchers, catchers	

Figure 4.1   Athlete Preparation Checklist

- Has read and understands testing procedures ____
- Has completed informed consent form ____
- Attended pretest training session ____
- Understands testing procedure ____
- Did not exercise the day of the test ____
- Ingested no food or beverages (other the water) for three hours before testing ____
- Has taken physician-required medications ____
- Is appropriately rested for testing ____
- Is wearing proper exercise clothing ____
- Is not feeling sick ____
- Has been properly and thoroughly warmed up ____

Facility and Equipment Preparation

The facility where the assessments are conducted can affect the quality of an athlete's performance, so it should be suitable for the purpose. Assessments should be administrated on appropriate surfaces that provide secure footing at all times. Ideally, the surface should be the same or similar to the surface used in the sport. For example, field turf is ideal for football, and a wooden floor is preferred for basketball. A challenge for the coach is to ensure that the environment does not affect performance. Elements such as wind, temperature, humidity, and so on should be controlled. An indoor facility is preferred.

Every coach is ethically responsible for providing a safe assessment environment. The assessment area should be spacious; speed assessments need a considerable distance for deceleration after the finish line. They should also be free of obstacles and hazards. To prevent accidents, the coach must make sure that athletes understand that assessments are no time for horseplay. Additionally, the atmosphere during the assessments should be controlled and private; spectators and other distractions should not be allowed at the facility because these can affect athletes' scores.

The coach should ensure that assessment administrators know which equipment to use and where it is located. The coach or the administrator should make sure that the equipment is on site and appropriately prepared before the assessment is scheduled to begin. The coach also needs to provide testing recording sheets, pencils, and clipboards and be sure that first-aid equipment and emergency procedures are in place.

Test Administration and Test Documentation

Assessment administrators should be properly trained in the application of the test and have a thorough understanding of all assessment procedures. If possible, they should administer the same assessments during each assessment period to ensure reliability and objectivity. If the same administrator is not available, the replacement administrator should have previously conducted assessments with the original administrator. An experienced assessment administrator should supervise a novice administrator to be sure all assessments are carried out and scored identically. Assessment consistency becomes even more critical in a pre- and postassessment analysis.

To administer a valid assessment with a high degree of reliability and objectivity, all of the elements of the assessment, including test supervision, warm-up, preparation, motivation, safety, number of assessment trials, and cool-down need to be considered. Properly planning and monitoring these elements produces a high degree of reliability in the testing and also maximizes the objectivity between assessment administrators, thus lessening the chance of erroneous results.

To facilitate proper test administration, the assessment administrator should develop a checklist (see figure 4.2) for each test (Graham 1994, Harman 2008). The administrator should always have access to a full description of the test protocols for reference. Additionally, all paperwork associated with the administration and recording of the test should be prepared before the testing session.

Speed assessments call for multiple trials, normally three, and the best score is recorded. The athlete should recover completely before performing subsequent assessments. Assessments that use high-intensity, short activities, which emphasise the phosphagen system, require 3 to 5 minutes for complete recovery. Therefore, assessments such as vertical jumps and the 30-yard dash can employ a multiple assessment battery. Every assessment session should conclude with a cool-down that includes static stretching. This is particularly important when the final assessment is one that stresses the lactic acid system, or is a high intensity, endurance activity, such as the 300-yard shuttle run. An adequate cool-down facilitates recovery.

Figure 4.2 Test Administration Checklist

- Test administrator is assigned and present for each test. ____
- Testing equipment is in working order and on site. ____
- Testing worksheet, pencils, and clipboards are distributed. ____
- Test administrators understand testing procedures. ____
- Location and time of tests has been organized. ____
- Test performance is clear to athletes and testers. ____
- Athletes are prepared for testing. ____
- First-aid equipment and emergency procedures are in place. ____
- All athletes are warmed up before testing. ____
- Atmosphere is controlled and private. ____
- Environmental conditions are acceptable and safe. ____
- Testing sites are spacious, clean, and ready. ____
- All athletes have cooled down after testing. ____
- Data analysis and evaluation responsibilities are set. ____

Sequencing

Although some coaches measure speed by itself, it is more common to assess speed within a battery of tests. When conducting multiple tests, appropriate sequencing is important. Test administrators should assess skills that require a high level of coordination and reaction before conducting tests that may cause fatigue and decrease performance (Graham 1994, Harman 2008). They should also conduct tests of explosive power and strength first because they require just 3 to 5 minutes of recovery time (Fleck 1983). Speed tests must be conducted early in a testing session and must take place after assessments that will cause fatigue. Proper sequencing maintains a high level of validity.

Athlete Preparation

In addition to completing the items on the Athlete Preparation Checklist (figure 4.1), on the day of the test, the administrator should give participants a thorough description of the test (this may need to be repeated to ensure full understanding) and one practice trial if possible (Graham 1994, Harman 2008). A warm-up that includes a movement preparation and dynamic activities precedes assessment day to prevent injury and maximize performance. Ideally, the warm-up is standardized for each testing session to help ensure reliability between sessions. A cool-down combining light exercise followed by stretching concludes every assessment to reduce the likelihood of muscle soreness.

Recording Scores

Coaches or assessment administrators should develop a scoring worksheet for the specific battery of tests to be given. Each assessment administrator needs a worksheet with an alphabetical list of athletes to be assessed at each station, along with space to record each trial and a best score. To ensure unbiased and accurate scoring, the assessment administrator or designated assistant is the only person recording scores at each assessment station. Athletes should not record or verbally provide assessment results.

NORMATIVE DATA

Speed and agility are important attributes for successful sport performance. Consequently, these performance parameters are included in most sport performance assessment batteries. What may be surprising is that normative data for athletic populations is often difficult to find. A simple explanation may lie in coaches' and strength and conditioning professionals' unwillingness to share results or provide valid, reliable, and objective data. Therefore, coaches and strength and conditioning professionals must often develop their own norms based on their own teams. Additionally, it is not uncommon for coaches and strength and conditioning professionals to develop their own assessment protocols that more closely mimic the requirements of their sport (e.g., 30-yard dash for baseball, 40-yard dash for football, 20-yard dash for women's softball).

Other factors that may limit the development of appropriate statistical data include protocol issues such as starting position (on the start line, 1 yard back from the start line) starting stance, (sideways, two-point or three-point stance), and timing method (handheld stopwatch or electronic timing device). When the aim of the program is to compare athletes' scores either before and after training or within the group (rather than compared to external norms), the protocol must be identical for each testing session rather than complying with an external protocol.

Because normative data for speed and agility assessment are limited, most norms are based on the cooperation of coaches in the specific sport. Through their support, percentile ranks have been established. Tables 4.2 to 4.6 provide normative data for speed testing for a variety of sports and athletes.

Table 4.2   High School Baseball

% rank	30-yard dash (sec.)	% rank	60-yard dash (sec.)
100	3.70	100	6.70
90	3.78	90	6.80
80	3.85	80	6.90
70	3.89	70	7.00
60	3.90	60	7.10
50	3.91	50	7.20
40	3.99	40	7.30
30	4.00	30	7.40
20	4.09	20	7.50
10	4.20	10	7.60

Adapted, by permission, from J. Hoffman, 2006, *Norms for fitness, performance, and health* (Champaign, IL: Human Kinetics), 110.

Table 4.3   Girl's High School Field Hockey

% rank	40-yard dash (sec.)	% rank	100-yard dash (sec.)
100	5.55	100	12.77
90	5.70	90	13.73
80	5.88	80	14.11
70	5.92	70	14.32
60	5.97	60	14.55
50	6.04	50	14.71
40	6.15	40	14.95
30	6.24	30	15.43
20	6.36	20	15.85
10	6.52	10	16.25

Table 4.4 Various Levels of Football

% rank	DB	RB	DL and OL	LB	QB	WR	TE
40-YARD DASH, MANUALLY TIMED (SEC.)							
Level: high school							
Position							
100	4.45	4.50	4.85	4.64	4.64	4.45	4.64
90	4.50	4.51	5.00	4.70	4.70	4.50	4.70
80	4.57	4.61	5.12	4.80	4.80	4.57	4.80
70	4.71	4.74	5.22	4.87	4.87	4.71	4.87
60	4.77	4.81	5.33	4.92	4.92	4.77	4.92
50	4.81	4.86	5.33	4.98	4.98	4.81	4.98
40	4.86	4.90	5.40	5.01	5.01	4.86	5.01
30	4.91	4.95	5.42	5.11	5.11	4.91	5.11
20	4.96	5.00	5.46	5.15	5.15	4.96	5.15
10	5.02	5.05	5.55	5.22	5.22	5.02	5.22

% rank	Manual	Electronic	Manual	Electronic	Manual	Electronic
40-YARD DASH (SEC.)						
	Level					
	14-15 years old	14-15 years old	16-18 years old	16-18 years old	NCAA D1	NCAA D1
100	4.75	4.96	4.60	4.87	4.49	4.68
90	4.86	5.08	4.70	4.98	4.58	4.75
80	5.00	5.17	4.80	5.10	4.67	4.84
70	5.10	5.28	4.89	5.21	4.73	4.92
60	5.20	5.31	4.96	5.30	4.80	5.01
50	5.28	5.43	5.08	5.40	4.87	5.10
40	5.38	5.52	5.17	5.46	4.93	5.18
30	5.50	5.63	5.30	5.63	5.02	5.32
20	5.84	5.84	5.45	5.73	5.18	5.48
10	6.16	6.22	5.73	5.84	5.33	5.70

Table 4.4 Various Levels of Football *(continued)*

	40-YARD DASH, MANUALLY TIMED (SEC.)							
	Level: college							
	Position							
% rank	DB	RB	DL	OL	LB	QB	WR	TE
100	4.34	4.44	4.72	5.07	4.57	4.60	4.42	4.66
90	4.41	4.50	4.80	5.15	4.62	4.70	4.46	4.78
80	4.48	4.55	4.87	5.21	4.66	4.75	4.50	4.80
70	4.56	4.60	4.90	5.25	4.72	4.79	4.55	4.83
60	4.63	4.63	4.93	5.30	4.76	4.81	4.60	4.90
50	4.70	4.67	4.96	5.33	4.78	4.86	4.67	4.96
40	4.75	4.74	5.03	5.40	4.81	4.91	4.72	4.99
30	4.79	4.80	5.09	5.47	4.86	4.99	4.77	5.02
20	4.83	4.85	5.15	5.56	4.92	5.06	4.80	5.07
10	4.86	4.88	5.21	5.61	4.97	5.13	4.84	5.11
	40-YARD DASH, MANUALLY TIMED (SEC.)							
	Level: NFL							
	Position							
% rank	DB	RB	DL	OL	LB	QB	WR	TE
100	4.30	4.40	4.67	5.02	4.51	4.55	4.34	4.61
90	4.34	4.44	4.72	5.07	4.57	4.60	4.42	4.66
80	4.41	4.50	4.80	5.15	4.62	4.70	4.46	4.78
70	4.48	4.55	4.87	5.21	4.66	4.75	4.50	4.80
60	4.56	4.60	4.90	5.25	4.72	4.79	4.55	4.83
50	4.63	4.63	4.93	5.30	4.76	4.81	4.60	4.90
40	4.70	4.67	4.96	5.33	4.78	4.86	4.67	4.96
30	4.75	4.74	5.03	5.40	4.81	4.91	4.72	4.99
20	4.79	4.80	5.09	5.47	4.86	4.99	4.77	5.02
10	4.83	4.85	5.15	5.56	4.92	5.06	4.80	5.07

Data from Hoffman (2006) and other sources.

Table 4.5 Boy's High School Soccer

% rank	40-yard dash (sec.)	% rank	100-yard dash (sec.)
100	4.72	100	10.76
90	4.90	90	11.62
80	5.01	80	11.79
70	5.11	70	11.97
60	5.16	60	12.05
50	5.23	50	12.38
40	5.40	40	12.59
30	5.49	30	12.87
20	5.67	20	13.38
10	5.88	10	14.00

Table 4.6 Girl's High School Multisport (Soccer, Softball, and Basketball)

% rank	40-yard dash (sec.)
100	5.55
90	5.70
80	5.88
70	5.92
60	5.97
50	6.04
40	6.15
30	6.24
20	6.36
10	6.52

TYPES OF SPEED ASSESSMENTS

Speed is measured as distance per unit of time and is typically identified as the time taken to cover a fixed distance. Assessments of speed are almost always conducted at distances less than 200 meters because longer distance reflects anaerobic endurance or aerobic capacity (based on the test distance) more than speed, and normally considerably shorter distances are used (Harman 2008). Speed tests can normally be categorized into two types depending on their starting mechanisms.

▶ **Static-start tests.** These are by far the most common tests and commence with an athlete in a stationary starting position. The 40-yard dash is probably the most recognizable speed assessment and commences from a static start. However, other speed assessments are gaining acceptance, probably because of their relevance to their specific sport (30- and 60-yard dash for baseball, 20- or 30-yard dash for basketball, 20-yard dash for softball). To provide the greatest test validity, coaches should determine what distances are typically run in the sport and select those distances for assessment.

Measuring split times provides additional information because this allows for an analysis of performance at different parts of a sprint. Timing gates set up at intermediate distances within the sprint can give the coach information about an athlete's strengths and weaknesses within each section of the overall distance. For example, if two athletes have identical 40-yard dash times, split times taken at 10, 20, and 30 yards can help differentiate what each athlete training needs. One may have great 10 and 20 yard splits but average 30 and 40 yard splits, revealing excellent accelerative ability but average ability at higher speeds. The other may have average 10 and 20 yard splits but great 30 and 40 yard splits, revealing average accelerative ability but excellent ability at higher speeds. The additional splits give a coach a more complete picture of each athlete.

▶ **Flying-start tests.** Most static-start tests assess an athlete's ability to accelerate. As mentioned in previous chapters, it can take a considerable distance for an athlete to reach maximum speed. Flying tests assess maximum speed by allowing a period of acceleration before the timed portion of the test starts. The start line is preceded by an acceleration zone, which needs to be long enough that the athlete can attain maximum speed before reaching it. Timing starts when the athlete breaks the start line and ends when he or she breaks the finish line. The distances should reflect the precise nature of the given sport.

40-YARD DASH FROM A STATIC START

Purpose

This assesses ability to accelerate.

Application

Forty yards is a commonly tested distance, but other distances should be selected to reflect typical sprints in the sport.

Equipment

Electronic timing device. (If a stopwatch is used, the assessor should start the watch on the first movement of the athlete's hand and stop the watch as the athlete's torso breaks the 40-yard line.)

Procedure

1. Athlete warms up and stretches.
2. Athlete takes two practice runs at submaximal speed for a specific warm-up.
3. Athlete stands behind starting line with one hand on the line on the start switch.
4. On the go command, the athlete accelerates over the test distance.
5. The athlete's torso breaks the light beam at the finish line to stop the clock. The athlete decelerates for 5 to 15 yards.
6. The best score of three trials is recorded to the nearest .01 second.

Variation

Place additional beams at 10 yards, 20 yards, and 30 yards to evaluate the athlete at these distances.

40-YARD DASH FROM A FLYING START

Purpose

To assess maximum speed capacity.

Application

Forty yards is commonly tested, but other distances should be selected to reflect the distances typically sprinted at maximum speed in other sports and the accelerative distance required to reach maximum speed.

Equipment

Electronic timing device. (If a stopwatch is used, the assessor should start the watch as the athlete's torso crosses the start line and stop the watch as the athlete's torso breaks the 40-yard line.)

Procedure

1. Athlete warms up and stretches.
2. Athlete takes two practice runs at submaximal speed for specific warm-up.
3. Athlete stands 30 yards behind the starting line.
4. On the go command, the athlete accelerates and reaches the start line at maximum speed.
5. The athlete's torso breaking the beam of light at the start line starts the clock and the torso breaking the beam at the finish line stops the clock. The athlete decelerates for 5 to 15 yards.
6. The best score of the three trials is recorded to the nearest .01 second.

Variation

Place additional beams at 10 yards, 20 yards, and 30 yards to evaluate the athlete at these distances. The acceleration zone can be adjusted according to the athlete's ability.

CHAPTER 5

Developing Sport-Specific Speed

Ian Jeffreys

The chapters to this point have outlined the scientific principles that contribute to speed, the technical requirements of running speed, methods of enhancing running speed, and guidelines for assessing speed. So far we have looked at speed as a general performance factor. However, the specific requirements for speed in sport are different between sports and even between positions within the same sport. This influences how speed training should be applied within a given sport. While we have alluded to these differences, the remainder of the book addresses developing speed in the context of specific sports. This allows coaches and athletes to develop speed in a way that benefits performance of the sport.

Developing speed that maximizes sport performance requires the development of several specific speed capacities and can be termed *gamespeed* (Jeffreys 2009). This allows the athlete to apply general speed capacity in a sport-specific setting, thus maximizing game performance, which is the ultimate aim of any training program. However, the basic abilities of accelerating and achieving high maximal running speeds still form the basis of an effective speed training program.

To ensure that speed improvements result in improved performance on the field of play, athletes and coaches must make subtle adaptations to the overall speed training program and use exercises that reflect the specific requirements of the sport. This can be thought of as applied practice and is conducted in addition to the basic speed development program. Developing sport-specific exercises requires a careful consideration of how speed is applied to specific sports and selecting and using exercise that apply speed in the same way.

This chapter outlines the processes for putting together sport-specific speed development programs. These processes can be used to develop a program for any sport. Chapter 6 provides sport-specific programs for many of the major sports, but if your sport is not covered, this chapter provides a system that can be used for any sport.

ANALYZING THE SPEED REQUIREMENTS OF A SPORT

Developing effective gamespeed requires an understanding of the sport in which an athlete needs to apply speed. Clearly, there are differences between sports, and this can be made even more complex by the differences between playing positions within the same sport. Additionally, with the massive range of activities that take place within field and team sports, analyzing speed application can be complicated.

While analyzing the speed requirements of different sports may at first seem a massive challenge, asking a few key questions can make the task much simpler. Working through the following questions will reveal a clear picture of the speed requirements of a specific sport, which in turn are addressed through a well-planned development program.

- ▶ What distances are typically run?
- ▶ In what direction does movement typically occur?
- ▶ What are the typical starting methods?
- ▶ What are the typical movement combinations?
- ▶ What stimuli trigger and control movement?
- ▶ How does speed relate to sort-specific skills and requirements?

These questions provide a framework on which to build a speed development program consisting of exercises and drills that maximize the transfer of basic speed qualities into sport-specific gamespeed.

TYPICAL MOVEMENT DISTANCES

Previous chapters have outlined the difference between maximum speed and acceleration and how these relate to the running distances involved. In sport, distances are often dictated by external factors, such as the court size in basketball and tennis, the rules regarding run and pass offense for offensive linemen in American football, and the distances between bases in baseball and softball. In these instances, it is relatively easy to identify typical distances of sprints. For other field sports such as soccer, it is not as straightforward because a host of distances must be covered, and many are position specific. However, even here, analysis that focuses on one player and his or her movement will reveal general patterns of movement distances. Analyzing the movement of most sports reveals a far greater reliance on acceleration than on maximum speed, so this should be reflected in the allocation of training time and effort spent on this aspect of performance.

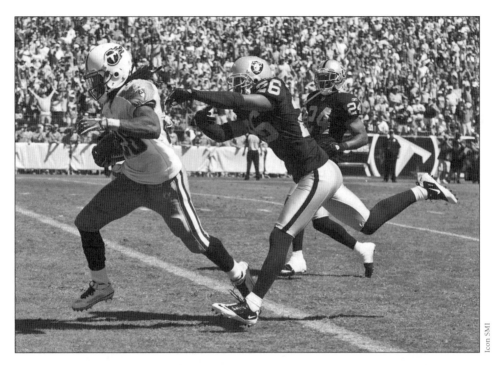

Running backs in American football like Chris Johnson accelerate and attain maximal speed over long distances to evade opponents and score touchdowns.

The analysis should include movement both on and off the ball. In many sports the vast majority of movement occurs off the ball, and this may involve different movement patterns than what are observed on the ball. In rugby, for instance, when on the ball, a scrum half's runs are predominantly short; however, watching off the ball reveals longer runs when in a supporting, or defensive covering, position. These patterns should be reflected in the allocation of sprint distances. These patterns also affect the role of maximum speed development. These longer distances and rolling starts may reveal that the player approaches and achieves maximum speed much more frequently than if on-the-ball movements had been analyzed in isolation.

TYPICAL MOVEMENT DIRECTIONS

Track sprinting is one dimensional in terms of its direction, simply requiring movement from the start to a finish 100 meters away, in a straight line. Most sports are not like this and require sprints in a multitude of directions. However, although it looks complex, once in motion, the multidirectional running action does not differ drastically from straight sprinting. What is critical is the ability to start in different directions and to change directions. These movements are termed initiation movements (Jeffreys 2007), and coaches can identify the typical directions in which an athlete will be required to sprint. Starting movement, for example, occurs in one of three predominant directions: to the front, to the side, and to the rear, with other directions being subtle variations of one of these types. Once an athlete has initiated movement in one of these directions, a more typical acceleration pattern takes place. Therefore, the ability to accelerate is fundamental to the vast majority of sports, with the major differences being the distance of acceleration and the actions following acceleration.

However, unlike the track sprinter, field and team sport athletes are unlikely to continue to accelerate in one direction. Instead, it is highly likely that they will be required to change direction at some point. In terms of direction change, two directions predominate: changing direction laterally or changing direction with an anterior or posterior emphasis. Careful analysis of sport movements reveals that multidirectional speed is simply a combination of these movement directions, and athletes armed with all of these abilities together with excellent accelerative and decelerative ability will be able to move effectively in multiple directions.

Another aspect of movement direction is the concept of curvilinear running. Many times an athlete's movement is not entirely straight, but makes subtle direction changes in response to the actions of the game. Here, direction changes are not sharp, but instead athletes run curved patterns, with the aim of maintaining running speed during this process. Analysis of the typical directions of movement in sport reveals where these curvilinear movement occur and in what typical combination of directions they occur. Speed in these curvilinear patterns can be developed by carefully selecting exercises that reflect this movement.

TYPICAL STARTING PATTERNS

Another key element of movement to ascertain is the initial starting position and especially whether starts are predominantly static (a batter at first base in baseball) or rolling (a tennis player coming forward into the net after a serve). Field sports differ greatly from track sprinting, where the sprinters start uniformly in blocks.

In reality, few team and field sports use a universal start pattern. Even where starts are static, these can vary in their set-up positions (standing square, standing staggered, or three point) and the initial direction of movement, which could be forward, lateral, to the rear, or a combination of these. Given these variations, athletes should master all of the typical starting scenarios they will face in a game. This can be achieved by varying the runs conducted in a training session.

While most traditional sprint training programs predominantly practice static starts, this may not allow full transfer to a game situation because in many sports speed does not usually initiate from a static start. Far more common are starts where an athlete is already in motion, what can be termed rolling starts. Here athletes already in motion need to accelerate in response to the requirements of the game unfolding around them. In sports where these actions are common, speed training needs to include these actions to develop an athlete's capacity to accelerate from a rolling start.

Rolling starts can vary in terms of their direction, their distance, and the preceding movement pattern. For example, soccer players accelerate while they are already in motion. However, while this movement could be linear, it could just as easily be in a multitude of directions, and the players could be shuffling or backpedaling before they accelerate. Subsequent acceleration, therefore, could be initiated from a range of preceding movement patterns. These initial patterns can vary in type and distance. To further complicate matters, the subsequent motion may require acceleration in a linear direction but could just as easily include acceleration laterally or to the rear. Clearly these variables add a sport-specific aspect to speed that needs to be practiced. Coaches and athletes should look at the typical patterns they need to produce in a game and integrate these into their speed training program.

Additionally, the purpose of the rolling start needs to be evaluated. In many instances, rolling starts are transition-based movements, which are movements that prepare the athlete for the main action. The athletes move while waiting to react to key aspects of the game. In this way they must be in a position that allows them to react quickly and effectively in response to a perceptual trigger from the game. Because the quality of the subsequent movement often depends on the quality of the transition movement, this movement should be practiced and mastered. Similarly, the associated movement combinations need to be practiced so the athlete can effectively carry out the movements required by the game.

Sport-specific speed training requires an analysis of the typical starting patterns. To facilitate this analysis, the following areas need to be looked at:

▶ **Static starts.** The essential components of static starts include the following:

- **Stance.** In general, a staggered stance in which one foot is placed ahead of the other is preferred because it places the athlete in a more effective acceleration position. This is the preferred stance if the athlete has a choice. However, in some instances, the sport dictates a square stance in which the feet are even with each other. If this is the case, the athlete should practice from this stance.

- **Subsequent movement direction.** Although subsequent movement is often linear, this is not always the case. For example, a baseball player at first base assumes a square stance to be able to see the pitcher and then accelerates laterally toward second base before turning to sprint.

▶ **Key variables of rolling starts.** Three key variables need to be ascertained.

- **Distance.** The distance of the rolling start affects the speed the athlete will achieve. If the rolling start is relatively long, the athlete will be able to attain a higher speed. In many sports a range of distances will be used, so rolling starts of different lengths should be practiced.
- **Direction.** The direction of the rolling start must be determined.
- **Typical movement patterns.** Once the typical patterns used in a rolling start (e.g., shuffling laterally) are identified, the athlete can practice the specific movement combinations to be able to accelerate rapidly from rolling the start.
- **Direction of subsequent motion.** Rolling starts may be predominantly linear, but they may also be multidirectional. Tennis, for example, requires rapid accelerations laterally from a split step or shuffle.

▶ **Rolling start as a transition.** Rolling starts may be used while an athlete is waiting to react to a stimulus. In this case, the focus of the rolling start should be on control and the quality of the movement after the stimulus, rather than speed.

TYPICAL MOVEMENT COMBINATIONS

The discussion of rolling starts leads naturally into a discussion of movement combinations. Seldom in sport does a burst of speed happen in isolation. Instead, it happens during the flow of a game, and is always preceded by either an initiation or transition movement (Jeffreys 2006a, Jeffreys 2006b). A task as simple as stealing second base can be broken into separate components: set up in a square stance, make a hip turn, accelerate, decelerate, and slide. In this instance, the movement combinations can be pieced together and practiced so that the whole movement becomes a well-honed skill. This is analogous to movements being joined together in a dance routine, with the quality depending on the individual moves and with the quality of how they flow into one another.

Even the most complex skills can be broken down so that typical movement combinations are identified, practiced, and developed. Here speed and agility intertwine and cannot always be separated, because sport performance requires an ever changing balance between these abilities. This is why it is sometimes best to look at sport speed training as movement training or gamespeed.

In this way, athletes are encouraged to demonstrate speed directly in the context of their sport. They must develop overall quality in a range of movement combinations and integrate this into a sport-directed speed training program. While traditionally, speed and agility have been seen as different aspects of performance, the reality is that in sport these need to be viewed as the same quality,

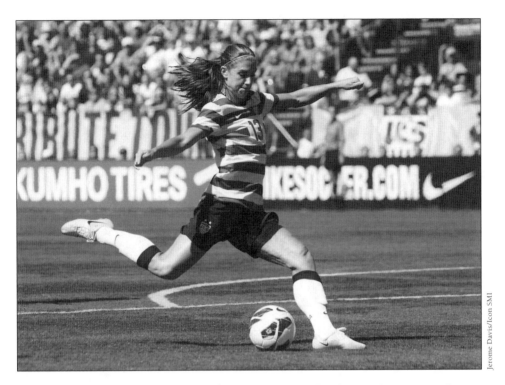

Alex Morgan combines speed and agility to beat defenders and set up goal-scoring opportunities.

with the aim to maximize performance through the application of movement that is of optimal speed and quality. For example, a basketball player trying to drive to the net may initiate a cut move to try to change direction and create space (agility) and follow this up with a rapid acceleration to the basket (speed).

The best athletes are the ones who can maximize their speed and agility performance and integrate them effectively into their sport-specific tasks. While basic speed provides an excellent basis for performance, unless it can be applied in the context of the sport and within the movement and skill requirements of that sport, it will never maximize performance. Here the concept of developing gamespeed is most useful, where the focus is on developing speed in a way that maximizes the transfer of speed to sport performance (Jeffreys 2009).

PERCEPTUAL STIMULI

Sport speed is nearly always triggered by an external stimulus. It is not uncommon to see athletes with better 40-yard-dash times being beaten to the ball by supposedly slower athletes who are able to move rapidly in the context of the game and in reaction to the game itself. Track sprinters often talk about moving on the B of the bang, with the gun providing an external, aural stimulus to trigger movement. This is a relatively simple stimulus and reflects the relatively

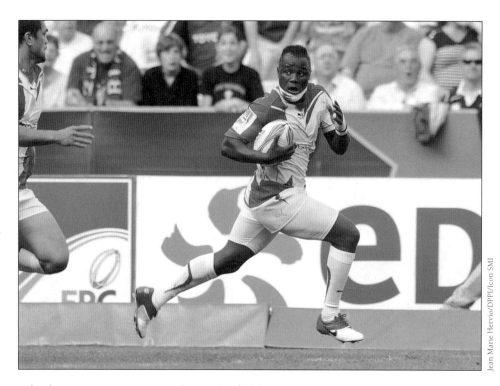

Jean Marie Hervio/DPPI/Icon SMI

Takudzwa Ngwenya sprints down the field, using the stimuli of the opponents and his teammates to direct his movements.

closed nature of track sprinting. In many sports, speed is triggered by a range of stimuli, both aural and visual. Basketball players, for example, react to the movement of the opposition, the movement of their teammates, and, obviously, to the movement of the ball. The nature and location of these stimuli provide the context for highly sport-specific speed training, where movement is triggered by a range of stimuli rather than simply starting on the "Go" or the whistle. As with all speed training, these abilities can be improved through training. However, care must be taken to ensure that these capacities are built on sound technical models (see chapter 3) and should not be introduced at the expense of the development of acceleration and maximum-speed techniques. Similarly, effective performance in the game situation should be built on a strength and power development program.

SPORT-SPECIFIC REQUIREMENTS

All the speed in the world is of no value if athletes cannot carry out the required sport skill when they get to their target area. This is paramount when planning a training program, and all technique development must enable the athlete to carry out the sport-specific requirements. To this end, it is important to integrate sport-specific requirements into training. Acceleration, for example, for a tennis player should involve the use of a racket, and any position attained must enable the player to play the required shot. In this way, elements such as balls can be integrated into the speed training session, providing a sport-specific practice.

Armed with the results of this analysis, coaches and athletes should be able to break down the specific speed requirement of a sport and identify key elements that need to be developed. The analysis should have identified fundamental patterns from which to construct programs that develop the athlete's ability through to sport-specific application. Chapter 6 provides advice from eight expert coaches on how to develop speed to enhance performance in specific sports. However, even if a sport is not covered in chapter 6, the information presented here should allow a coach or athlete to develop a sport-specific training program that can maximize the transfer of training directly into enhanced sport performance.

CHAPTER 6

Sport-Specific Speed Training

The chapters so far have outlined the fundamental factors influencing speed, the mechanical basis of speed, the key technical components of speed development, how to test for speed, and the principles for applying sport-specific speed training. In this chapter, leading experts describe how speed training can be applied to specific sports.

What is important here is not the exercises themselves but rather how to apply them to address a specific speed requirement of the sport. The coaches use the system outlined in chapter 5 to select exercises that will develop the specific speed requirements of the sport. It is important to note that the exercises are not necessarily sport specific as many exercises can be used across a range of sports. They focus on fundamental abilities such as acceleration, deceleration, and running at maximum speed, which are common to a multitude of sports, and therefore need to be developed appropriately. The programs use a range of basic exercises from chapter 3, and then once basic speed capacities have been developed, exercises that apply these in a sport-specific situation are used. Using this approach, coaches or athletes working in sports not covered in this section should be able to select exercises that address the speed requirements of their sport.

Sport-Specific Training for Speed

Sport	Page number
Baseball	90
Basketball	100
Football	115
Ice hockey	135
Rugby	145
Soccer	156
Tennis	170
Track	187

BASEBALL

Frank Spaniol

Speed never slumps is an adage often used in baseball. While it may seem an oversimplification, it is no secret that speed, both offensively and defensively, has a significant impact on baseball performance.

SPEED IN BASEBALL

For many years, the 60-yard dash has been used to test baseball speed and is considered the gold standard by many coaches and scouts. The average professional baseball player runs the 60-yard (55 m) dash in approximately 6.92 seconds. Outfielders are typically the fastest players, with an average time of 6.89 seconds, while infielders run an average of 6.97 seconds. Catchers are typically the slowest position players, with an average time of 7.19 seconds (Coleman and Lasky 1992; Spaniol 2007; Spaniol, Melrose, Bohling, and Bonnette 2005). The fastest position players typically are centerfielders, shortstops, and second basemen.

In addition to the 60-yard dash, some professional teams measure 30-yard (27.4 m) split times. Again, outfielders are the fastest position players, averaging 3.69 seconds in the first 30 yards and 3.20 seconds in the last 30 yards. Likewise, infielders average 3.73 seconds in the first 30 yards and 3.24 seconds in the last 30 yards, while catchers are the slowest with an average of 3.83 seconds in the first 30 yards and 3.36 seconds in the last 30 yards (Coleman and Lasky 1992).

IMPLICATIONS OF SPEED IN BASEBALL

While simple sprint speed can be useful in baseball, sport-specific speed is often a better indicator of success. One of the most common assessments of baseball-specific speed is the home-to-first base time, measured from the time the batter makes contact with the ball to the time he reaches first base. In the major leagues, the average right-handed batter reaches first base in 4.35 seconds, while the average left-handed batter reaches first base in 4.31 seconds. While the difference of .04 seconds may not appear significant, it actually equates to a left-handed batter reaching first base approximately 10 inches (25 cm) before a right-handed batter. Clearly, this can affect whether a player gets on base or is thrown out.

As in the 60-yard dash, outfielders are the fastest home-to-first runners, with an average time of 4.24 seconds (center fielder 4.16 sec., left fielder 4.30 sec., right fielder 4.29 sec.). Infielders are second fastest with an average of 4.36 seconds, with middle infielders averaging 4.27 seconds (shortstop 4.26 sec., second baseman 4.27 sec.) and corner infielders averaging 4.44 seconds (first baseman

4.50 sec., third baseman 4.39 sec.). The average catcher runs from home to first in 4.48 seconds (Coleman and Dupler 2005). So what do these running times mean? Are they significant in relation to baseball performance?

To answer these questions, let's look at the implications of a routine ground ball and subsequent close play at first base. The average centerfielder arrives at first base 2.10 feet (.64 m) ahead of a shortstop, 4.91 (1.50 m) feet ahead of a third baseman, and 6.82 (2.08 m) feet ahead of a catcher. The average shortstop arrives at first base .73 feet (.22 m) ahead of a right fielder, .80 feet (.24 m) ahead of a left fielder, 2.88 feet (.88 m) ahead of a third baseman, and 4.56 feet (1.39 m) ahead of a catcher. The average second baseman arrives at first base .52 feet (.16 m) ahead of a right fielder, .59 feet (.18 m) ahead of a left fielder, 2.68 feet (.82 m) ahead of a third baseman, and 4.34 feet (1.32m) ahead of a catcher (Coleman and Dupler 2005). Obviously, in a sport often referred to as "a game of inches," such differences are significant to the success of players reaching base safely and having a greater impact on their team's success.

Additionally, speed can have an important effect defensively. In the outfield, faster players can cover more ground in a given time. This allows faster players to make more plays, resulting in fewer hits for the opposition. In the infield, faster players may also be able to make more plays than slower players, improving a team's defensive scores. All this illustrates that speed can make an individual player better, and enhanced speed can improve a team's performance.

Based on these results, it is apparent that speed plays a vital role in successful baseball performance. Ironically, because of the short distances involved in the game, players rarely, if ever, achieve maximum speed (Cronin 2009). In actuality, it is acceleration that plays a much greater role in baseball than maximum speed because of the explosive starts and stops needed for success in the sport (Gambetta 2007).

FORCE AND SPEED

As outlined in chapter 1, Newton's second law of motion (law of acceleration) states that the acceleration of an object depends directly on the net force acting on the object and inversely on the mass of the object. Therefore, it is the ability of players to impart peak muscular and ground reaction forces, all in relation to their body mass, that contributes to greater relative acceleration (Cronin 2009). As the force acting on an object increases, the acceleration of the object increases. As the mass of an object increases, the acceleration of the object decreases. Therefore, when body mass goes up, acceleration goes down, unless force increases proportionally. Subsequently, a player's body composition plays an important role in acceleration, so when a player gains weight, every effort should be made to increase lean body mass (muscle), which has the potential to produce greater force.

In addition to improving force (strength), baseball players should also pay careful attention to appropriate body composition. The percent body fat for the average professional baseball pitcher is about 12.3 percent, catchers are 11.5 percent, infielders are 9.4 percent, and outfielders are 8.4 percent (Coleman 2000). Percent body fat for most college and high school players is slightly higher (Spaniol 2007, Spaniol 2005). To achieve maximum speed, baseball players should strive to maintain the optimal balance between lean body mass, fat mass, and force (strength).

BASEBALL-SPECIFIC DRILLS

While understanding the science behind speed in baseball is important, it is the practical application of that knowledge that is most critical for the player and coach. Therefore, it is imperative to use drills that train offensive and defensive acceleration and speed. Obviously, baseball performance requires quick acceleration based on a player's reaction to some type of external stimulus, usually a batted or thrown ball. From a defensive standpoint, players must train in an open environment, ready to react in any direction. The first drill trains this. Ball drops are excellent drills because they are easy to administer, are competitive, and train the stimulus–reaction–acceleration response that is so crucial to successful baseball performance.

From an offensive standpoint, base running requires powerful acceleration that transitions from a static base-running position (frontal plane), to a rotation or crossover step (transverse plane), then to a sprinting position (sagittal plane). The remaining drills are excellent for working on the transition to full acceleration (Coleman 2009).

Ball Drop

Aim   To develop the stimulus–reaction–acceleration response that is crucial for good defensive play.

Action   The drill uses tennis balls and a surface that is firm enough for balls to bounce at least twice. The player starts in a fielding position, which may be a square or staggered athletic stance, facing a partner or coach who is approximately 5 yards away. As the partner or coach drops the ball from shoulder height, the player explodes forward to catch the ball before it bounces twice. (The player should not dive unless the surface makes it safe to do so.)

Coaching Points

- The athlete initiates and maintains an acceleration posture on the ball drop.
- Arm drive is powerful, and the hand ranges from shoulder level in the front to a point behind at or just past the hip.
- The knee drives forward and up explosively while the other leg drives powerfully into the ground.

Variation   Difficulty can be increased by having the player move farther away from the partner or coach or by lowering the release point of the drop. Most players find it challenging to take a half or full step away from the partner or coach after each successful catch. The player can repeat the drill using a crossover step to the left, then a right crossover step. The drill can also be performed with the player's back to the partner or coach. The player turns, finds the ball, and catches it before it bounces twice. A variation that enhances the reaction–response component uses three partners or coaches positioned equal distances from the player (left, front, and right). They drop balls at random, requiring the player to react and accelerate in multiple directions, thus enhancing the reaction component.

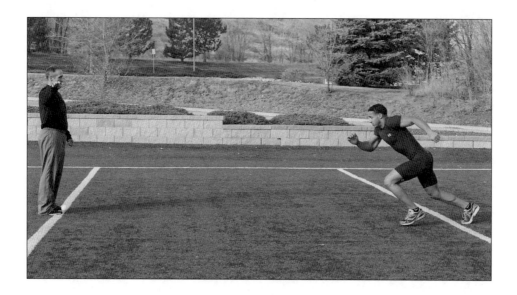

10-Yard Start

Aim To develop accelerative ability from a base-running stance.

Action The drill uses a starting line and a set of cones 10 yards away to mark the finish line. After an appropriate warm-up, the player starts in a base-running stance with the front foot on the start line (photo a). At a self-start or visual cue that requires the player to react (e.g., pitcher), the player rotates from the base-running stance to straight-ahead sprinting and accelerates through the 10-yard line (photo b). The coach times the sprint from the player's initial body movement until the runner crosses the 10-yard line. Players take two or three practice starts and then perform three to five runs for time. The athlete walks back and recovers for an additional 10 to 15 seconds after each run. An average time for this run is 2.0 seconds or faster, good times are 1.8 to 1.9 seconds, and an excellent time is less than 1.8 second.

Coaching Points

- An effective acceleration posture is initiated and maintained.
- Arm drive is powerful, and the hand ranges from shoulder level in the front to a point behind at or just past the hip.
- The knee drives forward and up explosively while the other leg drives powerfully into the ground.

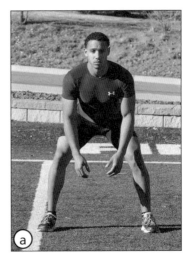

Base-running position.

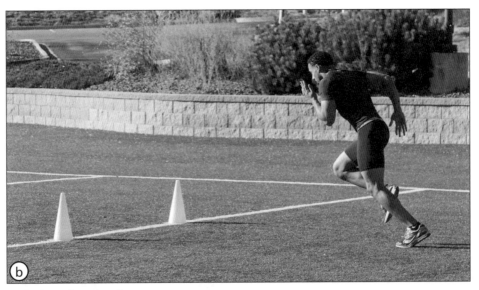

Sprinting after rotation.

30-Yard Sprint

Aim   To develop initial and transition accelerative ability.

Action   The drill uses two cones set up 30 yards apart. The runner starts at one cone, taking a base-runner lead, crossing over, and sprinting through the 30-yard mark for time (photos *a-c*). The watch is started on the first movement and stops when the runner crosses the second marker. The player performs two or three practice starts and then performs three to five runs for time. The athlete walks back and recovers for an additional 10 to 15 seconds. This is the approximate rest that they will receive on an aborted steal or a hit and run. An average time is 3.5 seconds or less. Good times are 3.3 to 3.4 seconds. An excellent time is less than 3.3 seconds.

Coaching Points

- Watch for the same acceleration posture, arm drive, and knee drive as for the 10-yard start.
- The athlete slowly shifts to a more upright running position.
- Perform an effective hip turn followed by an effective acceleration.

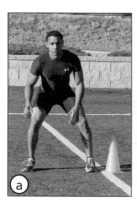 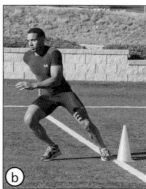 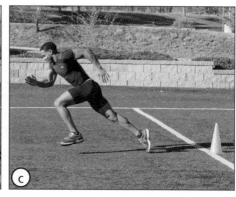

Curve Run (First Base to Third Base)

Aim   To develop the athlete's ability to sprint from first to third base. This is an important ability because offensive runs include this curved portion and considerable time can be lost through ineffective curve-running mechanics.

Action   This drill uses three cones set up 30 feet (about 10 m) apart on the warning track around the curve in the outfield from the right-field power alley to the left-field power alley. The first cone (start) is on the right-field side of center field, the second cone is in center field, and the third cone is on the left-field side of center field. The objective is to simulate going from first to third base. Runners take a base-runner lead and then a secondary lead (shuffle). From the secondary lead, the player crosses over, runs the outfield curve, and sprints through the third cone for time. The watch starts on the first movement and stops when the runner crosses the third cone. Players take two or three practice runs and then perform three to five runs for time. An average time is approximately 7.5 seconds. A good time is approximately 7.0 seconds. An excellent time is less than 7.0 seconds.

Coaching Points

- The athlete transitions from initial acceleration to high-speed running mechanics, becoming more upright in their running action in the process.
- The athlete maintains speed through the curve.
- The athlete leans into the curve while maintaining an effective posture.

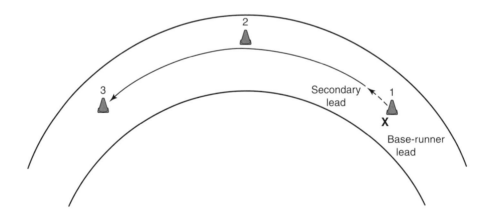

Curve Run (Home to Second Base)

Aim   To develop the ability to sprint from home to second base.

Action   The drill uses three cones set up 30 feet (about 10 m) apart on the warning track around the curve in the outfield from the right-field power alley to the left-field power alley. Cone 1 (start) is on the right-field side of center field, cone 2 is in center field, and cone 3 is on the left field side of center field. The objective is to simulate going from home to second base. The action is similar to the previous drill, but this time the player starts from a hitter's stance instead of a base-runner stance. The run is timed from the runner's first movement until the body crosses the third cone. Players take two or three practice runs and then perform three to five runs for time. Athletes walk back and recover for an additional 10 to 15 seconds. An average time is approximately 8.5 seconds. A good time is approximately 8 seconds. An excellent time is less than 8 seconds.

Coaching Points

- The athlete transitions from initial acceleration to high-speed running mechanics, moving from a low driving position to a more upright position.
- The athlete maintains speed through the curve.
- The athlete leans into the curve while maintaining an effective posture.

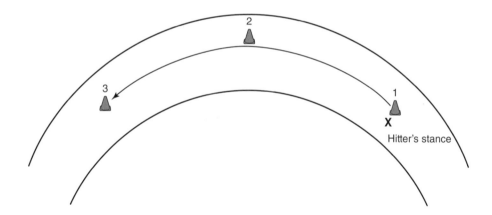

Ground-Ball Sprint

Aim   To develop the stimulus–reaction–acceleration response that is crucial for good infield defensive play.

Action   As the partner or coach hits a ground ball, the player accelerates forcefully to field it. The player starts in a fielding position facing home plate. The coach sets up in a batting position and hits ground balls toward the player. The difficulty can be increased by moving the player nearer the partner or coach. The coach or partner hits the ball in various directions and various distances away from the player. This requires the player to react and accelerate in multiple directions, thus enhancing the reaction component.

Coaching Points

- From the initial fielding position, the player initiates and maintains an acceleration posture.
- Arm drive is powerful, and the hand ranges from shoulder level in the front to a point behind at or just past the hip.
- The knee drives forward and up explosively while the other leg drives powerfully into the ground.

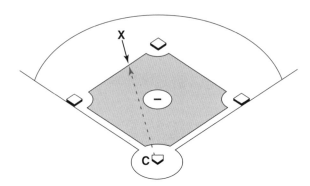

Fly-Ball Sprint

Aim   To develop the stimulus–reaction–acceleration response that is crucial for good outfield defensive play.

Action   As a partner or coach hits the fly ball, the player accelerates forcefully to catch it. The player starts in a fielding position, facing home plate. The coach sets up in a batting position and hits fly balls in the direction of the player. The player sprints to catch the ball. The difficulty can be increased by having the player cover a greater area. The coach or partner hits the ball in various directions and various distances away from the player. This requires the player to react and accelerate in multiple directions, thus enhancing the reaction component.

Coaching Points

- From the initial fielding position, the player initiates and maintains an acceleration posture.
- Arm drive is powerful, and the hand ranges from shoulder level in the front to a point behind at or just past the hip.
- The knee drives forward and up explosively while the other leg drives powerfully into the ground.

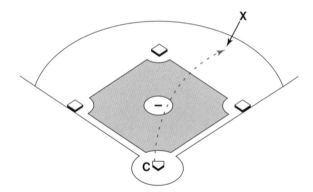

BASKETBALL

Al W. Biancani

Basketball is a speed sport, and, more specifically, it is an acceleration sport. This is largely dictated by the dimensions of the court: 94 feet by 50 feet. (International courts are 28 meters by 15 meters.) Subsequently, athletes must get to top speed as quickly as possible, making acceleration crucial to high performance both offensively and defensively. Even within this small court, most of the game is played in an even smaller area, the half court, so athletes have to beat their opponent to their respective positions on the floor in order to be successful in the game, thus making speed a vital commodity.

IMPLICATIONS OF SPEED IN BASKETBALL

Equally important to acceleration is an athlete's ability to exhibit this capacity within the basketball context. A look at the game clearly shows that while athletes do run forward, they also move backward, laterally, and on a curved plane. For example, they often must switch from a defensive position into a full-speed sprint, or they run backward and in a split second have to accelerate forward as fast as possible.

During offensive plays, athletes may fake one way then reverse direction and sprint to another spot on the floor. An example is an offensive athlete who makes a V-cut at the top of the key, reverses direction, goes around a pick, and then sprints to the opposite corner to receive the ball. Here the path is a curved pattern. At the same time, defensive athletes need to demonstrate effective speed and movement capability in order to track these offensive movements. Defensive athletes' success is determined by their ability to stay with their assigned person; therefore, speed and effective movement are important commodities.

Within the game, perhaps the greatest expression of basketball speed is during a fast break where one athlete breaks out in front of everyone to shoot a layup while a defender must try to keep up at all times. Clearly, athletes who improve their speed give themselves a distinct advantage in terms of enhancing the quality of their play.

DEVELOPING BASKETBALL SPEED

The previous examples of the demonstration of speed in basketball provide a basis on which to develop a basketball speed program. Athletes accelerate from both standing and rolling starts to high speed on both offense and defense in order to perform their required assignments. These plays require that speed be manifested in many directions over various distances and from a variety of starting positions and speeds, and thus need to be practiced. Additionally, speed is often expressed as a reaction to an opponent's movements, a teammate's movements, or the movement of the ball, and it is also expressed both on and off the ball. Offensive players need to be able to dribble the ball while sprinting, emphasizing how speed and fundamental sport skills are intricately linked.

BASKETBALL-SPECIFIC DRILLS

Because the ability to accelerate quickly is clearly required, many teams test their athletes for half-court speed. A good time is 1.8 to 2.3 seconds depending on the position played. By developing proper running mechanics and improving acceleration, athletes can improve their half-court time by .1 to .2 seconds, which is significant for this distance. Despite this, many basketball players use poor running mechanics, limiting their speed potential. The initial drills in this section teach running mechanics and acceleration, work on quick hands and feet. Additional drills apply these abilities in a basketball context.

Running Mechanics

Effective sprint mechanics ensure that both the force and the resulting acceleration are in the forward direction, maximizing speed. Good sprint mechanics must be emphasized and maintained at all times. The four components of sprint mechanics important to basketball are arm action, hip action, body lean, and running stride effectiveness (length and cadence). The following drills develop proper running mechanics.

The athlete must understand the importance of the arm action in running speed. In simple terms, the arms govern the legs: the faster an athlete can swing the arms efficiently, the faster the legs will move, enabling higher speeds and rates of acceleration. Effective arm movement includes loose and relaxed shoulders, an efficient forward and backward arm swing, appropriate arm bend, and comfortable hand position.

The first component of proper arm movement is arm swing. The emphasis is on keeping the shoulders down and relaxed so the arms can swing freely. The arms essentially move forward and back in a straight line and not excessively across the body. Excessive motion across the body causes the shoulders to move from side to side and results in upper-body forces contrary to straight-line running. Keeping the arms close to the body and sliding the arms against the shirt helps develop this action.

Once the swing is developed, coaches can teach the appropriate arm angle. The athlete bends the elbows to a 90- to 105-degree angle and swings the arm from the shoulder, focusing on moving the arms forward and back in a straight line. The elbow angle does not change excessively. Releasing the arm angle excessively decreases leverage power and diminishes corresponding leg drive. The hands should not move past the hips on the backswing and should never go higher than the chin or shoulder on the forward action. Athletes can practice these techniques in front of a mirror so they can self-correct their arm action.

Arm action is closely linked to leg action. Effective leg action is the ability to drive the leg forward through the hips and then cycle the leg through to enable a subsequent action. This requires hip strength and mobility. Tight hips limit the ability to fully flex the knee, which shortens the stride, provides less drive, and ultimately hinders sprint speed.

Sprinting is a rhythmical losing and gaining of one's balance. Proper body lean is crucial in maximizing the efficiency of this phenomenon. The running stride can be broken down for teaching and training purposes into three drills or the ABC drills: high knee lift (A drill), foreleg reach with active pull-back (B drill), and back leg extension (C drill). The A and B drills develop the technical aspects of maximal speed. However, their use with more senior athletes is limited because athletes at this level should focus on the application of speed to basketball, which requires more acceleration-based exercises. The drills that focus on running mechanics can be performed every day as part of the warm-up.

Seated Arm Swing

Aim   To develop an effective arm action.

Action   The athlete sits on the ground with legs extended and pumps the arms quickly, imagining each hand is hitting a bongo drum positioned at hip height. "Beating the drum" encourages quick, powerful arm action. The harder the arm comes back, the harder the opposite leg pushes backward to the next step. When proper arm action and force are applied the athlete slightly bounces off the ground. The elbow angle should not change much during the drill.

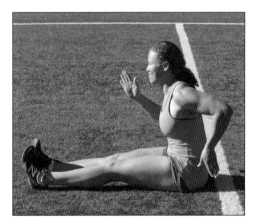

Coaching Points

- Emphasize the drum at the hip and keeping the arm as close to the torso as possible by sliding on the shirt.
- Remind players that arm action is important because arm speed governs leg speed.
- Hands should come to shoulder level on the upswing and the hip on the backswing.

Fall Forward

Aim   To develop proper posture during acceleration.

Action   The athlete stands on the balls of the feet, with the arms at the side of the body and bent, ready to run with the first step (photo *a*). From this start position, the athlete falls forward with a whole body lean into the first step of a run (photo *b*). The body naturally assumes the proper body lean on the first step: The torso is held as straight as possible, as if there were a line from the head to the ankles and a feeling of being tall.

Coaching Points

- The aim is to keep a straight line posture.
- The knees are driven powerfully forward and up.
- The arms are driven powerfully to supplement the knee drive.

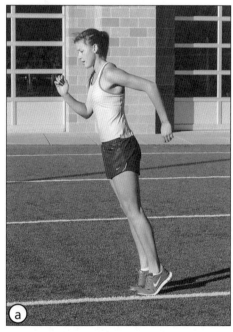

a

Forward lean.

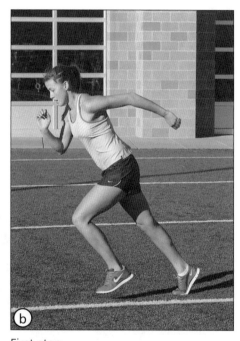

b

First step.

High Knee Lift (A Drill)

Aim   To develop the knee lift during front-side mechanics.

Action   The athlete faces forward and stands as tall as possible. The athlete marches forward, raising the knee of the lead leg so that the thigh is about parallel to the ground on each step, and the supporting leg remains straight. The athlete stays on the ball of each foot and pushes up as the other knee rises. The foot on the lifted knee leg is flexed and positioned directly under the raised knee. The drill is carried out for a given distance, such as 10 meters, or for a given time, such as 4 to 6 seconds.

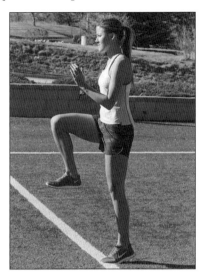

Coaching Points

- Emphasize a rhythmic and fluid raising of the lead leg through a good range of motion.
- Emphasize the foot behind the knee and emphasize why the bottom leg should be straight.
- Emphasize staying tall.
- Proper arm action must be emphasized.

Variation   To increase the difficulty, the player lifts the knees high while skipping. This can also be performed for distance or for time. Another variation is high-knee running. Players move down the court or field at a run, taking about three steps per meter.

Foreleg Reach With Active Pull-Back (B Drill)

Aim   To develop the reach and cycle elements of sprint mechanics. The skipping and running versions of this drill strengthen the hamstring and gluteus muscles.

Action   The athlete stands on one leg, raises the knee of the other leg, extends the lower leg, and paws the foot back to the ground (active pull-back). The heel then comes up toward the buttocks, and the whole action is repeated with the same leg (photos a-d). This can be performed for distance, about 10 yards, or for time, about 4 to 6 seconds. An active pull-back emphasizes pawing the ground and bringing the heel to the buttocks. The follow-through of the flexed ankle and heel moving to the buttocks positions the leg and foot to repeat the drive movement quickly and efficiently. The athlete repeats the drill on the other leg. Once the athlete can consistently perform the movement correctly, continue the exercise using the appropriate sprint arm drive.

Coaching Points

- Instruct the athlete to lead with the knee before extending the lower leg. The active pull-back positions the foot so that it can push into the ground. According to Newton's third law, the harder the athlete pushes against the ground, the harder the ground pushes back, sending the runner forward.

- The pawing foot should land near the grounded foot in order to maximize the pushing force. If the foot hits the ground too far in front of the athlete, less force can be applied and the athlete loses momentum and power.
- Effective arm action should be emphasized.

Variation The athlete performs the motion while moving forward, initially marching, then skipping. Athletes can progress to running with a high knee lift, a good foreleg reach, and an active pull-back. Focus is on the active pull-back, or pawing, motion during this variation. The athlete's movement down should be slow, with an emphasis on maintaining body lean. The upper body should be ahead of the athlete's center of gravity, and each step should be onto the balls of the feet rather than flat-footed.

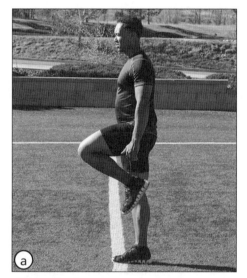

Lifting the knee.

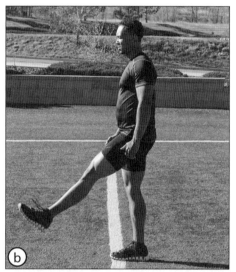

Extending the lower leg.

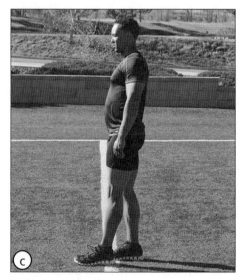

Pulling back.

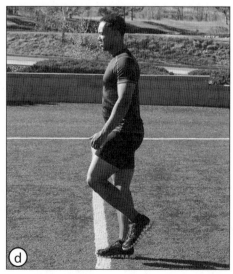

Lifting the foot.

Back-Leg Extension or Bounding (C Drill)

Aim To develop the drive action and emphasize back-side mechanics.

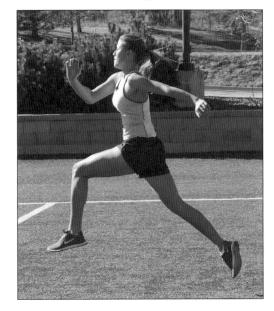

Action The athlete drives the body forward as powerfully as possible, using the driving action of the leg. The athlete should have a high knee lift and a full extension of the drive leg.

Coaching Points

- Encourage as much hang time as possible.
- Focus on full back-leg extension and pushing off with the toes.
- Emphasize knee drive.
- Utilize a powerful proper arm action at all times. This can be either a double arm drive where both arms drive forward and back at the same time or an action which is an exaggerated action where arms drive alternatively forward and back.

Variation The athlete completes the action while skipping, with an emphasis on getting high in the air, driving the lead knee up, and pushing off with the support leg into full extension. Next, the athlete can bound from one leg to the other. Emphasis is on the back-leg extension. The lead knee drives up and remains up as the opposing back leg achieves a full push or extension. Athletes should aim to cover as much distance as possible on the bounding variation.

Butt Kick

Aim To develop effective mechanics during the recovery phase of the stride. Flexibility and good back-kick recovery allow for a greater range of motion and can lengthen an athlete's stride.

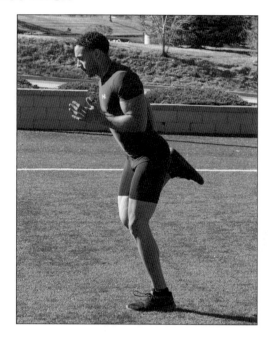

Action The athlete runs while bringing each heel up toward and touching the buttocks if possible. The arms are bent, swinging loosely from the shoulders, and pulling the hand back toward the hip (like beating a drum). Although athletes tap the heel to the buttocks as fast as they can, forward progression is slow because each step is small.

Coaching Points

- The range of motion behind the body should be limited, as if a wall exists behind the athlete.
- Emphasize a fluid range of motion.

Figure Eight

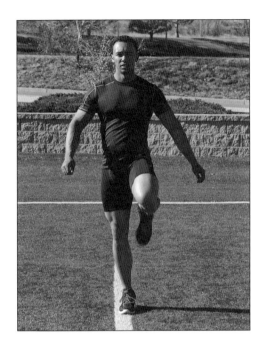

Aim   To develop hip mobility.

Action   The athlete walks forward, overemphasizing the movement of the hips in a vertical figure-eight motion. The pelvis rolls forward to achieve the fullest range of motion. Once the athlete can consistently perform the movement correctly, continue the exercise using the appropriate sprint arm drive.

Coaching Points

- The movement should be fluid.
- The hip movement should occur without any compensatory movements in the upper body.

Acceleration

Given the small dimensions of a basketball court and the short distances covered during a game, acceleration is a key component of successful basketball performance. The ability to accelerate can be developed initially through general drills, but as players become more competent in these abilities, basketball-related exercises allow players to apply the acceleration capacities they have developed directly into enhanced game performance. The four drills that appear after the running-mechanics drills help players improve their acceleration capabilities:

- ▶ Four step
- ▶ Shuffle and accelerate
- ▶ Quick arm and foot
- ▶ Resisted running

Four Step

Aim   To develop the ability to accelerate quickly by gradually lengthening the stride during the transition from a static position to a full sprint.

Action   Tape or some other marker indicates the starting line and the distances for the four steps. Step 1 is 30 inches (about 75 cm) from the starting point, step 2 is 40 inches (about 100 cm) from step 1, step 3 is 50 inches (about 125 cm) from step 2, and step 4 is 60 inches (about 150 cm) from step 3. The athlete stands at the starting position and starts running through the four steps at quarter speed, avoiding hesitation between the first and second step. One foot lands just inside each measured step marker. The athlete should initially start in a low driving position and then gradually rise to a more upright position.

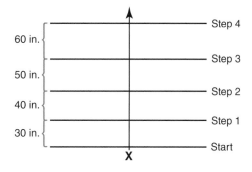

Coaching Points

- Emphasize that the first four or five steps in an athlete's start are crucial and should be executed with explosive power.
- Focus on an initial arm drive that creates an explosive first step.
- Emphasize an arm movement that beats back to the hip. The harder the arms are pumped, the harder the opposite leg will drive.
- Emphasize a quick arm action; arm speed governs leg speed.
- Encourage athletes to think of their steps as if they are a four-speed transmission.

Variation   The initial focus is on technical development rather than on maximum speed. Progression can involve graduating to three-quarter effort and then to 100 percent effort. This technique can be thought of as a smooth transition (like a drag car with a four-speed transmission). As the athlete becomes proficient at accelerating, add a ball to develop the important speed–skill link.

Shuffle and Accelerate

Aim   To develop the athlete's ability to accelerate from a lateral movement.

Action   The drill uses three cones set up in a straight line, with 5 yards between cones. The athlete side shuffles between cones 1 and 2 and then accelerates through a four-step acceleration to cone 3.

Coaching Points

- Remind athletes to maintain an athletic position throughout the shuffle.
- Emphasize that the first four or five steps in an athlete's start are crucial and should be executed with explosive power.
- Focus on the initial arm drive to create an explosive first step.
- Emphasize driving the leg forward and up to maximize acceleration.

Variation   The acceleration drill can be performed from various starting movements, for example, backpedaling and then accelerating. The combinations practiced should reflect those deployed in a game. Initially, the drill can initiate from a self-start. Later an external stimulus can be added to trigger movement.

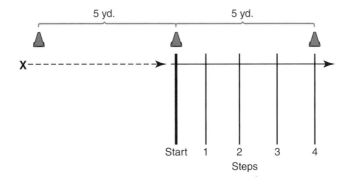

Quick Arm and Foot

Aim   To improve both arm and foot speed and promote a smooth acceleration from standing still to running.

Action   The coach sets up flat pieces of wood, plastic, or tape to mark a starting point and lines (or rungs) progressively farther apart. The first rung is 18 inches (about 45 cm) from the starting line; the second is 24 inches (about 60 cm) from that line. Additional lines are at 30 inches (about 75 cm), 36 inches (about 90 cm), 42 inches (about 120 cm), and 48 inches (about 120) from each preceding line. Next the coach sets up 10 low hurdles 48 inches (about 120 cm) ahead of the last line. Hurdle heights of 3, 5, or 7 inches (about 7.5, 13 or 18 cm) can be used. Athletes begin with the 3-inch hurdles and increase the height as comfort and mastery are achieved. The 3-inch hurdles are set up 48 inches (about 120 cm) apart, the 5-inch hurdles 54 inches (about 135 cm) apart, and the 7-inch hurdles 60 inches (about 150 cm) apart.

The athlete accelerates through the floor markings, emphasizing rapid leg turnover using a fast-hands, fast-feet action as if going through a speed ladder. The athlete immediately sprints through the 10 hurdles, taking two steps between hurdles. Athletes should repeat the drill so they lead with both legs. Before putting the whole drill together, athletes may need to practice simply running through the spaced hurdles. They should begin by running through the line by stepping with one foot between the hurdles and progress to completing two steps between the hurdles. Running between the hurdles with two feet down requires very quick arm movement.

Coaching Points

- Explain that the distance between rungs and hurdles is deliberately shorter than normal acceleration and running strides to develop quick hand and foot movements.
- Emphasize a smooth, quickstep acceleration.
- Focus on moving through the rungs using fast feet and hand movements. Quick arms are crucial. Emphasize that quick arm action governs quick leg action.
- Emphasize proper running mechanics at all times.
- Focus on proper acceleration technique.
- Focus on maintaining speed through the 10 hurdles.

Variation Drills can be done both with single leg and double legs between hurdles. The following two variations provide good workouts for this drill, but these can be modified depending on need.

- Variation 1: 10 runs over 10 3-inch hurdles only with no acceleration component. Slowly walk back to the start to recover.
- Variation 2: Include the acceleration component.
  - 5 runs over 10 3-inch hurdles
  - 5 runs over 10 5-inch hurdles
  - 5 runs over 10 7-inch hurdles
  - Slowly walk back to the start to recover

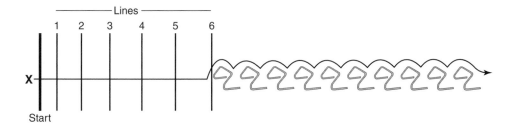

Resisted Running

Aim   To develop a driving action.

Action   A variety of methods can be used to provide resistance: sleds, parachutes, and so on (see chapter 3). For this drill, heavy-duty tubing is placed around an athlete's waist and a partner behind provides resistance. The athlete sprints a given distance, pumping the arms back hard toward the hip, emphasizing good form throughout the distance. As advised in chapter 3, resistance should be relatively low to ensure that the athlete's sprint technique is not negatively affected.

Coaching Points

- Focus on the initial arm drive to create an explosive first step.
- Emphasize driving the leg forward and up to maximize acceleration.
- Maintain an effective acceleration posture throughout.
- Effective arm action must be emphasized throughout.

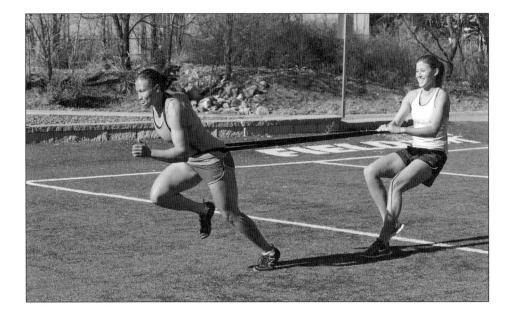

Accelerate and Decelerate

Aim   To develop the ability to accelerate and then rapidly decelerate to defensive position.

Action   The drill uses two cones set up 5 yards apart. The athlete starts by standing in a defensive position at one cone. The athlete accelerates rapidly forward toward the other cone and then decelerates to a stop before reaching it (photos *a* and *b*). The athlete assumes a defensive position immediately on reaching the cone.

Coaching Points

- Focus on the initial arm drive to create an explosive first step.
- Emphasize driving the leg forward and up to maximize acceleration.
- Remind athletes to shorten the strides, lower the center of mass, and widen the distance between the feet as they approach the second cone.

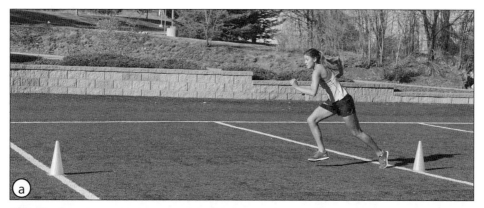

Sprinting.

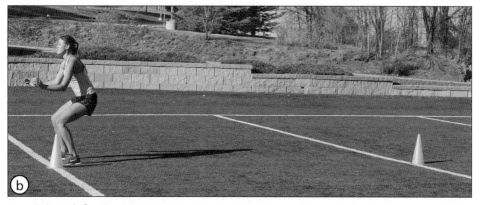

Regaining defensive position.

Drive Past

Aim   To develop offensive acceleration to beat an opponent.

Action   The athlete stands in a triple-threat position on or near the three-point line with a partner standing 1 yard away directly in front. From this position the athlete accelerates with a dribble past the opponent for a layup or dunk.

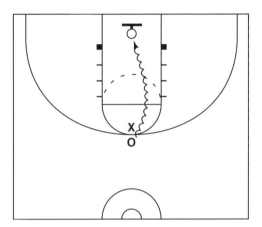

Coaching Points

- The athlete uses a rapid first step, and dribbles the ball in the hand away from the opponent.
- The athlete assumes an effective acceleration posture.

Variation   This drill can become progressively more competitive by having the defender make greater attempts to stop the offensive player from getting past. This requires the offensive player to make stronger attempts to outwit the defender and create the space for the drive past.

Give-and-Go Acceleration

Aim   To develop the ability to accelerate in a game-specific context.

Action   The athlete stands 2 yards outside the three-point line with a ball. A partner stands 3 yards inside the three-point line. The athlete passes the ball to the partner and immediately accelerates toward the basket. The partner then passes the ball to the athlete, who attempts a layup or dunk.

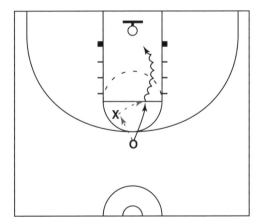

Coaching Points

- Athletes focus on rapid acceleration.
- Remind athletes to adjust their feet and body position to receive the pass while maintaining speed and to adjust their actions appropriately to score the basket.

FOOTBALL

Jeff Kipp

Football is a diverse sport played by a variety of athletes, whose ideal physical stature is largely dictated by the requirements of each playing position. However, one common thread provides an advantage for all football players at any position: to be faster than the opponent. It has been said that in football strength punishes, but speed kills. Speed training for football can be as complex or as simple as the coaching staff chooses to make it. It is not necessary to go out and spend a lot of money on specific equipment. Even though the requirements for playing speed depend on position, every athlete on the field can benefit from training to become faster.

SPEED IN FOOTBALL

In football, like in most field sports, speed is not merely a linear measure, and getting from point A to point B as fast as possible is not the only important variable. The ability to take a powerful first step in any direction is critical in maximizing playing speed. Additionally, players need to be able to move quickly, putting their bodies in an advantageous position for a subsequent movement such as acceleration, deceleration, or changing direction. Regardless of position, it is essential for a football player to have the capability to move laterally as efficiently and quickly as possible.

An athlete's speed and agility can be facilitated by their ability to recognize what is happening and react quickly and appropriately to the stimulus. The ability to reaccelerate after a reaction or change of direction or both is important for the athlete to be able to gain as much ground as possible or to limit the opponents' ability to gain ground.

IMPLICATIONS OF SPEED IN FOOTBALL

The precise nature of speed application varies among playing positions. The following information explores several important considerations.

First-Step Acceleration

Training the first step or developing an explosive first movement in a linear, or forward, direction teaches an athlete to overcome inertia and move the center of mass from a stationary position as quickly and explosively as possible. The goal is for the athlete to learn the body position and the correct angles, including positive shin angle, to produce the most explosive movement possible.

Football players use a lateral or angled first step more often than a straight-ahead movement. This step must be explosive and quick. From the offensive side of the ball, an explosive first step can create leverage and position when blocking, as well as create an advantage against the pursuing defense. On defense, an explosive first movement can make the difference in being blocked or avoiding the block. It can eliminate the advantage the offense has in knowing the play. The drills presented later teach the athlete the correct body position and explosive movements required for an efficient first step in any direction.

Acceleration

The athlete's ability to accelerate is a key component of football and should become a primary component of training. Acceleration is the rate of change of velocity, and the aim of training is to increase the rate at which an athlete can increase running speed, resulting in achieving maximum speed in a minimal amount of time.

Deceleration

An often overlooked training area for a football player is deceleration. Coaches throw athletes into change-of-direction drills without considering whether or not they are prepared to withstand the forces associated with deceleration and change of direction. To minimize the potential for injury during these movements, coaches should consider the alignment of the athlete's lower-body limbs and joints. Preparing an athlete with adequate deceleration training before introducing change-of-direction drills contributes to more efficient and effective changes of direction during the agility drills and on the field. Football is played in all directions; therefore, a training regimen should target many different directions and angles of acceleration and deceleration.

Recognition and Reaction

It is prudent for the coach to assist the athletes in developing recognition and reaction abilities in their training. Football players' ability to recognize what is happening around them and to react quickly and efficiently plays heavily into the success or failure of their respective functions on the field. Recognition and reaction components can be woven into the drills that develop speed to save time and make drills more complex. Most athletes slow during a drill in which they are required to think and react.

The goal of recognition-and-reaction training in combination with a drill is to bridge the gap between the athlete's top speed in a given drill and their slower speed when required to react to a stimulus. Expensive lighting and timing systems can provide this stimulus, but simple visual signals with a hand, ball, or body movements or auditory signals by a coach are simple and effective ways to add stimulus to any drill. Also, these signals can be developed to reflect the perceptual stimuli an athlete needs to react to in a game.

Drills that incorporate recognition-and-reaction training can range from simple to complex. A ball drop, where the athlete must react to the ball's movement and catch it before it bounces twice can be a simple, stand-alone drill. Exercises in which an athlete maneuvers through an agility drill and then reacts to a single step by a coach or teammate add a decision-making component to the drill. These drills can also be varied according to positional requirements. A running back, for example, reacts in a direction opposite to the stimulus to avoid a tackle; whereas, a linebacker reacts in the same direction as the movement to simulate following the play.

Maximum Speed

Although football is a game of angles, leverage, acceleration, and change of direction, all players can benefit from training their top or maximum speed. Although the amount of ground covered and the opportunity for full-speed running is largely position specific, developing maximum speed can be beneficial. (Review the discussion of maximum speed in chapter 2 for more on the benefits.) Training at or near maximum speed may not be the primary focal point of the training in football, but it should certainly be an area of consideration.

FOOTBALL-SPECIFIC DRILLS

Choosing the appropriate drills for the team's situation and constraints can provide challenges for the football or strength and conditioning coach. Variables such as space, time, personnel, age, experience, and training level of the athletes all play a part in program design and exercise selection. Choosing a clear focus for the training session can narrow the choices and help the coach design a pointed and effective training session.

A simple method to separate training focuses is to divide the program into a linear portion and a multidirectional portion. Developing linear speed uses exercises targeting straight-ahead movements like the forward start, acceleration, deceleration, and top-speed running. The multidirectional portion takes into account the development of an explosive start in any direction, along with subsequent acceleration, deceleration, and change of direction. Classifying exercises and drills into one of these categories can help the coach define the focus of the training.

It is also important to take into account the level of training of the athletes. Most athletes start with basic movements to gain a solid foundation for future training. All athletes should then follow a logical progression to assure their readiness for additional stresses and more difficult or complex movements. Some athletes will progress to more advanced movements faster than others, and variety may be needed within sessions to account for this.

This section provides drills that develop speed in a football context. Individually, each exercise means little, but when taken together and with the effective manipulation of variation, volume, and intensity, they complete the bigger picture (see table 6.1). The overall training program needs goals and a plan to achieve them. This plan should spell out the goal of the training and use exercises, volumes, variable intensities, and recovery to assist the coach and team in attaining their goals.

Table 6.1 Sample Planning Grid

Dates	Dec. Week 1-4 Postseason/transition	Jan. Week 5-8 Off-season 1	Feb. Week 9-12 Off-season 2	Mar. Week 13-16 Spring training	Apr. Week 17-20 Off-season 3	May Week 21-24 Off-season 4	June Week 25-28 Off-season 5	July Week 29-32 Off-season 6	Aug. Week 33-36 Preseason/fall practice	Sep.-Nov. Week 37-49 In season
EXERCISES										
Single-leg box explosion (single response)		3 × 4-6 (each leg)				3 × 4-6 (each leg)				
Single-leg box explosion (multiple response)			3 × 4-6 (each leg)				3 × 4-6 (each leg)	3 × 4-6 (each leg)		
Even-stance broad jump (single response)	3 × 4				3 × 4					
Even-stance broad jump (multiple response)		3 × 4				3 × 4				
Hopping even-stance broad jump		2 × 4				2 × 4				

Dates	Dec. Week 1-4 Postseason/transition	Jan. Week 5-8 Off-season 1	Feb. Week 9-12 Off-season 2	Mar. Week 13-16 Spring training	Apr. Week 17-20 Off-season 3	May Week 21-24 Off-season 4	June Week 25-28 Off-season 5	July Week 29-32 Off-season 6	Aug. Week 33-36 Preseason/fall practice	Sep.-Nov. Week 37-49 In season
EXERCISES										
Uneven-stance broad jump (single response)	3 × 3 each				3 × 3 each					
Hopping uneven-stance broad jump		2 × 4				2 × 4		3 × 3-4 (each leg)		
Lateral broad jump (single response)	3 × 4 (each leg)				3 × 4 (each leg)					
Lateral broad jump (multiple response)		2 × 4 (each leg)				2 × 4 (each leg)				
Hopping (one-leg take off; land on the opposite foot) lateral broad jump			4-6 (each leg)				4-6 (each leg)			
Lateral quarter-squat push-off (balance)	3 × 4 (each leg)				3 × 4 (each leg)					

(continued)

Table 6.1 Sample Planning Grid *(continued)*

Dates	Dec. Week 1-4 Postseason/transition	Jan. Week 5-8 Off-season 1	Feb. Week 9-12 Off-season 2	Mar. Week 13-16 Spring training	Apr. Week 17-20 Off-season 3	May Week 21-24 Off-season 4	June Week 25-28 Off-season 5	July Week 29-32 Off-season 6	Aug. Week 33-36 Preseason/fall practice	Sep.-Nov. Week 37-49 In season
EXERCISES										
Lateral quarter-squat push-off (multiple response to balance)		3 × 3-4 (each leg)				3 × 3-4 (each leg)				
Lateral quarter-squat push-off (reaction and multiple response to balance)			3 × 3-4 (each leg)				3 × 3-4 (each leg)	3 × 3-4 (each leg)		
Angled quarter-squat push-off (balance)	3 × 4 (each leg)				3 × 4 (each leg)					
Angled quarter-squat push-off (multiple response to balance)			3 × 3-4 (each leg)				3 × 3-4 (each leg)	3 × 3-4 (each leg)		
Hurdle shuffle (move laterally over 3 hurdles and return)	3 × 4 (each leg)									
Hurdle shuffle (double response)	4 each				4 each					

Dates	Dec. Week 1-4 Postseason/transition	Jan. Week 5-8 Off-season 1	Feb. Week 9-12 Off-season 2	Mar. Week 13-16 Spring training	Apr. Week 17-20 Off-season 3	May Week 21-24 Off-season 4	June Week 25-28 Off-season 5	July Week 29-32 Off-season 6	Aug. Week 33-36 Preseason/fall practice	Sep.-Nov. Week 37-49 In season
EXERCISES										
Hurdle shuffle (triple response)		4 (each leg)				4 (each leg)				
Hurdle shuffle (single return)		2 (each leg)				2 (each leg)				
Hurdle shuffle (double return)			2 (each leg)				2-4 (each leg)			
Hurdle shuffle (triple return)								2-4 (each leg)		
Hurdle shuffle to forward sprint			3 (each leg)				3 (each leg)			
Wall drive (position hold)	2 × 3 (each leg)				2 × 3 (each leg)					
Wall drive (tap)	2 × 6 (each leg)				2 × 6 (each leg)					
Wall drive (march)	3 × 6 (each leg)				3 × 6 (each leg)					
Wall drive (single response)	3 × 8	3 × 8			3 × 8	3 × 8				
Wall drive (double response)		3 × 4 (each leg)	3 × 6 (each leg)			3 × 4 (each leg)	3 × 6 (each leg)			
Wall drive (triple response)			3 × 6				3 × 6	3 × 6		

(continued)

Table 6.1 Sample Planning Grid *(continued)*

Dates	Dec. Week 1-4 Postseason/transition	Jan. Week 5-8 Off-season 1	Feb. Week 9-12 Off-season 2	Mar. Week 13-16 Spring training	Apr. Week 17-20 Off-season 3	May Week 21-24 Off-season 4	June Week 25-28 Off-season 5	July Week 29-32 Off-season 6	Aug. Week 33-36 Preseason/fall practice	Sep.-Nov. Week 37-49 In season
EXERCISES										
Wall drive (rapid)			2 × 5 sec.					2 × 5 sec.	3 × 5 sec.	
Mountain climber (single response)	3 × 8	3 × 8			3 × 8	3 × 8				
Mountain climber (double response)		3 × 4 (each leg)	3 × 6 (each leg)			3 × 4 (each leg)	3 × 6 (each leg)			
Mountain climber (triple response)			3 × 6				3 × 6	3 × 6		
Mountain climber (rapid)			2 × 5 sec.					2 × 5 sec.	3 × 5 sec.	
Falling start (6 yards)	6				6					
Falling start (10 yards)		6				6				
Falling start (15 yards)			6				6	6		
Ins and outs		3	5			3	5	6-7		
Four-cone square agility (focus on the quality of the movement patterns in each section)	2-3 (each leg)									

122

Dates	Dec. Week 1-4 Postseason/transition	Jan. Week 5-8 Off-season 1	Feb. Week 9-12 Off-season 2	Mar. Week 13-16 Spring training	Apr. Week 17-20 Off-season 3	May Week 21-24 Off-season 4	June Week 25-28 Off-season 5	July Week 29-32 Off-season 6	Aug. Week 33-36 Preseason/fall practice	Sep.-Nov. Week 37-49 In season
EXERCISES										
Four-cone square agility		2-3 (each leg)			2-3 (each leg)	2-3 (each leg)		2-3 (each leg)		
Zigzag agility (focus on the quality of the movement patterns in each section)	2-3 (each leg)									
Zigzag agility		2-3 (each leg)			2-3 (each leg)	2-3 (each leg)		2-3 (each leg)		

General suggestions for designing the program include dividing speed work into linear and lateral training days (see tables 6.2 and 6.3), beginning with simple, easy-to-coach drills and exercises progressing to more complex and challenging exercises. Plyometric exercises also play a role in a speed training program, and these can progress from two-leg movements to single-leg movements and from single-response exercises to multiple-response exercises. If speed and power are the goal, full recovery is recommended.

Table 6.2   Sample Plan for Linear Speed and Acceleration

Week 5, day 1, Jan. 1-7

The focus is on linear first step and acceleration. Athletes start at exercise group 1 and progress sequentially through to group 6.

Group 1	Group 2	Group 3
Warm-up 20 jumping jacks 20 crossover jacks 20 cross-country skier 20 split jacks	Dynamic flexibility 1 lunge 5 body-weight squat 5 each inverted hamstring 5 each knee hug/quad stretch 5 inchworm	Build-up 2 × 25 yards at 50% 2 × 25 yards at 75% 2 × 25 yards at 100%
Group 4	**Group 5**	**Group 6**
Speed technique 3 × 8 wall drive (single response) 3 × 4 each wall drive (double response) 6 × 10-yard falling start	Explosive training 3 × 4 single-leg box explosion (single response) 2 × 4 each uneven-stance broad jump 2 × 4 hopping broad jump	Cool down/stretch 10 min. rope stretch

Table 6.3   Sample Plan for Lateral Speed

Week 5, day 2, Jan. 1-7

The focus is on lateral speed. Athletes start at exercise group 1 and progress sequentially through to group 6.

Group 1	Group 2	Group 3
Warm-up 5 min. jump rope (various)	Dynamic flexibility 5 each lateral lunge 5 each crossover lunge 5 each Spiderman 5 each leg cradle 5 each straight-leg march	Build-up 2 × 25 yards side skip 2 × 25 yards crossover run 2 × 25 yards at 100%
Group 4	**Group 5**	**Group 6**
Lateral movement 4 each hurdle shuffle (triple response) 2 each hurdle shuffle (single return) 2 × 3 each lateral quarter-squat push-off (multiple response to balance)	Agility 3 each four-cone square agility 3 × zigzag agility	Cool down/stretch 10 min. foam roller

Single-Leg Box Explosion

Aim To develop linear first-step speed and acceleration.

Action The athlete places one foot on a 6- to 15-inch (15-38 cm) box (or stadium step or bleacher) while remaining in a hip-width stance. The shin of the leg on the box is parallel to the torso and supporting leg. The arms are in a loose, 90-degree position, with the arm opposite the leg on the box in a forward blocked position (photo a). Assuming a position to the side of the box lets the athlete retain a forward lean while keeping the feet hip-width apart and allows the athlete to drive off of the box without fear of landing on the box. With the foot on the box, the athlete pushes off and forcefully drives the opposite knee upward, maintaining dorsiflexion (toes toward shin) at the ankle and driving the body as high as possible. During the movement, the athlete drives the arms into opposite positions, maintaining the loose 90-degree angle at the elbows. The majority of arm movement occurs at the shoulder joints (photo b). The athlete should be able to perform the movement without bending at the waist or allowing the back to hunch over.

Coaching Points

- The back is flat and the eyes are on the horizon.
- The knee drives and the hips do not move backward.
- Remind athletes to move as explosively as possible from a stationary position without performing a countermovement.

Variation The athlete begins with a low box to develop coordination during the exercise, then increases the height to build strength though a greater range of motion. This movement more closely resembles the height of the knee drive while running. Additionally, the athlete progresses from single-response sets to multiple or continuous response sets. To add specificity, the athlete can react to visual or auditory commands.

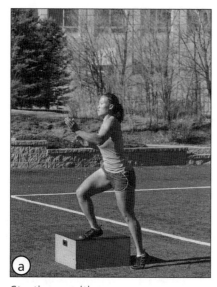

Starting position.

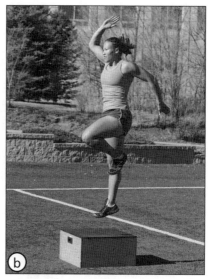

Dorsiflexion of the ankle and driving the other knee.

Broad Jump With Even and Uneven Stance

Aim To develop linear first-step speed, acceleration, and deceleration.

Action The athlete assumes an athletic, or ready, position. The knees and hips are slightly flexed and the feet are in complete contact with the ground. The weight is shifted slightly forward, creating pressure on the ball of the foot (photo a). Athletes use the even stance until they are comfortable with the exercise and have learned to explosively move the hips and center of mass forward. When athletes have become proficient, they can use the uneven stance, and the goal is to push off of both legs and not just one. For the even stance, the athlete should use a hip-width or slightly wider foot position, with the feet side by side. For the uneven stance, the athlete also uses a hip-width or slightly wider foot position, but one foot is slightly behind the other so that the toes of that foot are even with the heel of the other foot.

From either starting position, the athlete jumps, driving the hips forward as far as possible (photo b). On reaching full extension at the hips, knees, and ankles, the athlete pulls the heels toward the butt, creating a cycling motion with the feet and dorsiflexing the ankle joint (toes toward shin). The athlete then flexes the hips, driving the knees forward and bringing the heels through (photo c). The athlete should "stick" the landing without the use of an extra hop or step to regain balance. To practice being in a good starting position for subsequent movements, the landing position resembles the even athletic stance, and the athlete should not collapse into a deep squat.

Coaching Points

- Athletes jump off the whole foot, focusing on the ball of the foot, to use the larger muscles of the quadriceps and glutes and minimize the absorption of force at the ankle.
- The back is flat, chest up, and head in a neutral position with the eyes focused 5 to 10 yards ahead, not looking at the feet.
- Remind athletes to jump off both feet and not to collapse on the landing.

Variation This drill can be made more difficult by adding one or two 6-inch (15 cm) hurdles for the athlete to jump over. A further progression for this drill is to have the athlete begin the drill by hopping in place (ankle hops) and then jumping, thus increasing the use of the stretch-shortening cycle. The coach can introduce reaction and recognition by having the athlete bounce and then jump only when a visual or auditory command is given. Additional variations can include the lateral broad jump. This version can be performed from an even or uneven foot placement to simulate the playing environment. The athlete should still take off and land on both feet.

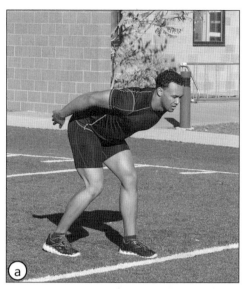

Starting position with uneven stance.

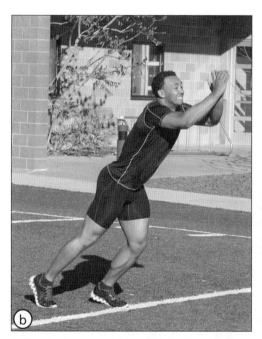

Full extension and hips forward.

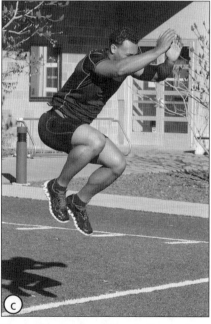

Knees forward and heels through.

Lateral or Angled Quarter-Squat Push-off (Balance)

Aim   To develop lateral first-step speed, lateral deceleration, and change of direction speed.

Action   The athlete begins the drill in a quarter-squat position with the thighs just above parallel to the ground. The knees are bent, the hips are back, and the chest is up. The feet are slightly wider than hip width, giving the athlete a solid base. From the quarter-squat position, the athlete pushes off one leg (trail leg) and moves laterally, landing on the opposite foot (lead leg). This exercise can be performed using lateral or angled movements. On landing, the athlete sticks the landing and resumes the position of the lead leg to the quarter-squat position. The hips are back and even. Athletes may try to balance by moving the hips and trail leg, but they should try to limit this movement to improve balance and technique.

Coaching Points

- Athletes push laterally off of the whole foot with a focus on the ball of the foot to use the larger muscles of the quadriceps and glutes and minimize the absorption of force at the ankle.
- The back is flat, chest up, and head in a neutral position with the eyes focused 5 to 10 yards ahead, not looking at the feet.
- Athletes stick the landing and don't collapse or use an extra hop or step for balance.

Variation   The difficulty can be increased by adding one or more 6-inch (15 cm) hurdles for the athlete to move over. Once the correct body position can be maintained, the athlete may progress to multiple-response repetitions (several actions performed repeatedly). These can initially be in the same direction and then varied to develop to a change-of-direction response (for example, a sprint in the opposite or an angled direction, a turn and run, a backpedal). Reaction and recognition can be introduced by having the athlete move only when a visual or auditory command is given. As the athlete performs the movement, a coach may throw a reaction ball or tennis ball in front of the athlete, requiring reaction and pursuit.

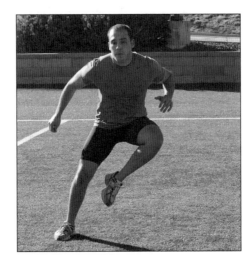

Wall Drive

Aim   To develop acceleration technique.

Action   The athlete leans forward against a wall (or a railing or partner) with the arms extended and the palms of the hands flat against the wall. Hips and knees should be fully extended. The athlete raises one leg so that the hip and knee are both flexed to about 90 degrees. Keeping the upper body still, the athlete drives the flexed, or drive, leg down so that the hip and knee are extended. Simultaneously, the athlete drives the trail leg up so that the hip and knee on that leg flex to 90 degrees, and the ankle remains dorsiflexed. The athlete has essentially switched legs quickly and powerfully in a single action. (This is the single-response version.)

Coaching Points

- The hips are forward, head neutral, and chest up.
- The heel of trail leg on the ground, and the foot is flat with pressure on the ball of the foot.
- The hips do not shift backward during the drill.

Variation   To simplify the movement, the athlete can start by alternating legs: right knee up, then both feet down, then left knee up, holding each position for 15 seconds. The athlete progresses to a single-leg tap, in which the lead leg drives down to tap the ground next to the trail leg and immediately returns to the knee-drive position. The athlete can then march while holding the correct body position.

The athlete can move to the single-response version already described. To increase the difficulty, the athlete can use a double response (where two actions are performed consecutively ending up in the same start position), a triple response (three actions performed consecutively), and finally a rapid fire for a set time (usually just 5 seconds). Finally, the athlete can take one arm off the wall and swing it in a loose 90-degree position to train it along with the legs.

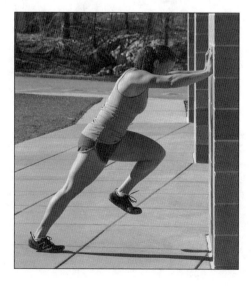

Mountain Climber

Aim   To develop acceleration technique.

Action   The athlete assumes a push-up position with hands and toes on the ground and the arms extended, the back flat, and the knees and hips extended. Then the athlete flexes one leg at the knee and hip and positions that foot on the ground under the hips. The hips do not rise away from the ground. This is the start position. On the coach's command, the athlete drives the lead leg back to a fully extended position and moves the extended leg forward to the bent-knee and bent-hip position (photos *a* and *b*). The hips should not bounce or rise during this movement.

Coaching Points

- The back is flat, head neutral, and hips and knees fully extended.
- Remind athletes to focus on extending the drive leg directly to the fully extended trail-leg position.
- Athletes switch both legs at the same time and keep the drive knee between the arms.

Variation   To simplify the movement, the athlete can first learn the positions through this sequence: right knee forward, both legs straight, and left knee forward. The athlete holds each position for 15 seconds. The athlete can then march while holding the correct body positions. At this point, the athlete is ready for the single-response version already described. This drill can move forward to a double response (switch and return), a triple response (switch, return, and switch) and finally a rapid fire for a set time, usually about 5 seconds.

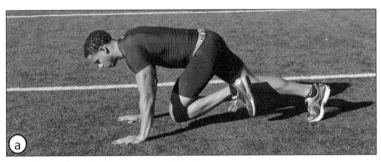

One knee forward.

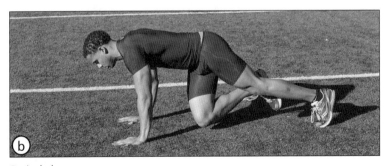

Switch legs.

Falling Start

Aim   To develop acceleration and first-step explosion.

Action   The athlete begins in a tall standing position with the feet directly under the hips, chest up, head neutral, and eyes focused straight ahead. The athlete falls forward, maintaining a straight line with the hips forward (photo *a*). The athlete does not bend at the waist or hips and does not round the back. The athlete falls as far as possible before forcefully flexing the hip and knee of the drive leg to 90 degrees at both the knee and hip and drives the arms in the opposite positions from the legs (photo *b*). The drive leg continues into a first step by driving the hips forward explosively while maintaining the straight-line posture. This step is followed immediately by an explosive second step while maintaining the posture. The athlete does not perform the drill at full speed until mastering the correct form. The athlete performs the drill using the natural drive leg and then using the other leg. The athlete needs to be able to take an explosive first step with both leg.

Coaching Points

- Keeping the body straight and tall, the athlete falls as far as possible before initiating the drive leg.
- The chest is up throughout the movement, and there is no bend at the waist or rounding of the back.
- Remind athletes to explosively drive the leg and drive the hips as far forward as possible.

Variation   After athletes master the first two or three steps using proper technique, they can progress to a more explosive start and carry out the drill for 5 to 10 yards. They may also perform the drill on a slight uphill (2-3 degrees) or slight downhill or a combination of uphill, downhill, and flat.

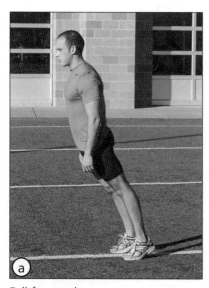

Fall forward.

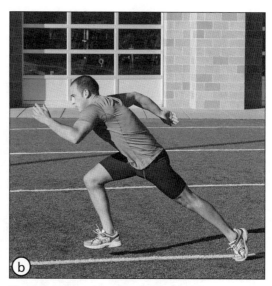

Flexing hip and knee of drive leg.

Ins and Outs

Aim To develop linear speed and speed endurance.

Action The athlete begins in a two-point start stance. On the coach's signal the athlete sprints for about 60 yards using the following pattern. Through the first 20 yards, the athlete builds up to about 75 percent speed, keeping a forward lean and a positive shin angle. The head stays in a neutral position with the face and shoulders relaxed. From 20 yards to 30 yards, the athlete sprints full speed. From 30 yards to 40 yards, the athlete strides out, attempting to maintain speed and body position. From 40 yards to 50 yards, the athlete runs full speed again, and then strides out from 50 yards to 60 yards. (If using a court, the athlete may only be able to run at full speed for one 10-yard interval.)

Coaching Points
- The athlete maintains positive shin and body position.
- The arms are at a loose 90-degree angle.
- Remind athletes not to reach for steps.

Variation The drill can be varied by changing the distance for the build-up and the other intervals (e.g., 25 yards for build-up, 15 yards for full speed, 15 yards for stride)

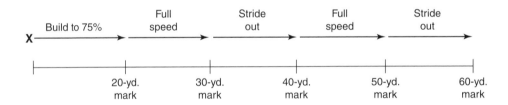

Four-Cone Square Agility

Aim   To practice combining acceleration, deceleration, and change of direction.

Action   The coach sets up four cones in a square so the corners are 5 yards apart. The athlete begins in an athletic, or ready, stance with the feet a little wider than hip width, knees bent, hips down, chest up, back flat, and head in a neutral position. The athlete begins at the first cone in the ready position and powerfully accelerates toward the second cone. The athlete uses a deceleration step and stop, balancing on the outside cutting leg. The athlete holds this position for a moment and then resets into the ready position by cone 2. The athlete shuffles from left to right. The athlete again sticks the outside cutting leg and balances for a moment before resetting into the ready position. The athlete backpedals from cone 3 to cone 4 and again sticks and balances on the outside leg. The athlete resets and then shuffles from cone 4 back to cone 1.

Coaching Points

- The athlete bends the knees and sits into the decelerations, keeping the back flat and the head neutral.
- The player drives off of both feet to jump out of the pattern changes.
- The stance does not become too wide during the changes. If the stance is too wide or the outside knee is not bent enough, power diminishes from that leg causing a less explosive movement out of the turn.

Variation   To simplify the drill, it can be broken into linear sections, focusing on the deceleration and the drive coming out of the turn. To increase difficulty, athletes perform the drill as fast as possible while maintaining good body, hip, knee, and ankle position at the turns. Recognition and reaction work can be added to the drill by using a ball drop after one of the cones or a reaction to another person's movement. Introducing competition by timing the drill can add stimulus and improve speed.

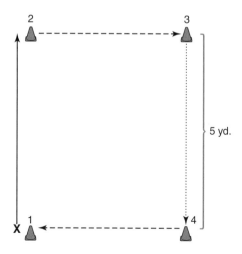

Zigzag Agility

Aim   To practice acceleration, deceleration, and change of direction.

Action   Five cones are set up approximately 5 yards apart in a zigzag pattern. The athletes begin the drill in an athletic, or ready, stance. At cone 1, the athlete takes an explosive step in the direction of the cone 2 and accelerates to cone 2. The athlete breaks down at cone 2, using a deceleration step and an outside cut step. The athlete sticks the outside cut step and balances. The athlete pushes off of the outside cut step and drives toward cone 3. The athlete breaks down again using only a deceleration step and an outside cut step. The athlete repeats this process through the rest of the cones.

Coaching Points

- The back is flat and head neutral.
- The hips drive toward the target, and the athlete does not reach out with the foot for the next step.
- After balancing on the outside cut leg, the athlete drives off as hard as possible toward the next cone.

Variation   Progression can be provided by moving faster through the cones and spending less time balancing on cuts until the movement is continuous. The coach can also lengthen the distance between cones or space them closer. Athletes can also run inside the cones using an inside or speed cut, like rounding a base in baseball.

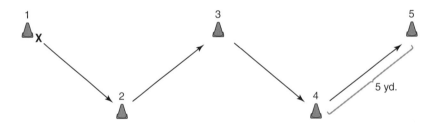

ICE HOCKEY

Mark Stephenson

Ice hockey has been referred to as the fastest game in the world. Whether this is true or not, it is undoubtedly a game of speed and quickness played on an area no bigger than 100 feet by 200 feet (about 30 m × 60 m). In a typical phase of play in ice hockey, a player may skate all out for 30 to 45 seconds, requiring bursts of speed and acceleration and abrupt changes of direction (Manners 2004). An improvement in an athlete's speed may increase performance (Warren, McDowell, and Scarlett 2001).

However, ice hockey is different from the other sports covered in this book because speed in ice hockey does not refer to running speed. Instead it refers to skating speed. Therefore, many of the technical points made in the early chapters together with the drills based on running mechanics have far less value in ice hockey. Indeed, there is little research that suggests that enhancing running speed will increase skating speed. This is a good example of the specific nature of speed, which has been discussed extensively elsewhere.

SPEED IN ICE HOCKEY

Although running speed is not a major concern for ice hockey players, speed training should be an essential part of their strength and conditioning program. As in most other sports, enhanced speed can give an ice hockey player an advantage in both offensive and defensive situations. One principle common between running speed and skating speed is that strength training is critical in developing speed and acceleration. Therefore, a major portion of speed training for ice hockey should develop the strength and power characteristics required for effective skating performance. This should focus on developing the explosive-strength capacities of the leg musculature responsible for the skating motion.

Strength and conditioning training for ice hockey can take place both on and off the ice. Incorporating various on-ice speed training methods with off-ice conditioning, such as strength training and plyometric training, will develop speed to enhance overall performance. Off-ice conditioning should focus on developing key physical capabilities, while on-ice conditioning should focus on speed and the endurance and agility capabilities specific to hockey. Depending on the periodization model being used, the majority of off-ice physical development usually occurs during the off-season, although a degree of off-ice work should continue throughout the season to maintain the player's strength and power. Off-ice work can be especially useful when ice access is limited.

Whether speed development is on ice or off ice, several factors need to be addressed. Speed training involves explosive power, and therefore, should only be performed when the body is fully recovered (Lentz and Hardyk 2005). Adequate rest between bouts allows the athlete to perform at full capacity and with proper technique. A work-to-rest ratio of at least one to four is recommended. Training tips for developing explosive speed are summarized here:

▶ Perform speed training at the beginning of the workout.

▶ Use a one to four work-to-rest ratio between repetitions.

▶ Perform all work at 90 percent of full velocity or higher.

▶ When using resistance, allow no more than a 10 percent decrease in velocity.

▶ Incorporate drills that move both linearly and laterally.

Although running speed may not be crucial for ice hockey players, athletes can still apply many of the concepts for developing running speed. In many of the sprint drills, players and coaches can substitute skating for running. Similarly, drills that train key movement combinations can also be used to develop on-ice speed. Additionally, on-ice training can incorporate resisted drills, such as those that use elastic bands, to provide an overload to the drive phase of acceleration.

IMPLICATIONS OF SPEED IN ICE HOCKEY

While speed is not the only factor affecting successful ice hockey performance, improved speed can offer a great advantage to any player, both offensively and defensively. Players with greater speed get to the puck faster, enhancing the opportunity to maintain or win possession and providing more time to make effective game-based decisions. Offensively, greater speed offers an enhanced attacking threat, enabling a wider choice of attacking options. Defensively, greater speed provides a potent defense against a range of attacking threats.

ICE HOCKEY–SPECIFIC DRILLS

These exercises supplement a basic strength and conditioning program to produce physical adaptations that will increase ice hockey speed. They are divided into two categories: on-ice conditioning and off-ice conditioning. The on-ice work is speed specific, and the off-ice conditioning develops the key physical characteristics that enhance on-ice speed.

On-Ice Conditioning

The aim of speed development for ice hockey players is to improve their speed on the ice. This allows them to express speed directly in the playing of the game, providing a potential advantage both offensively and defensively. Therefore, speed training must reflect the requirements of the game. Chapter 5 provides guidelines for determining the speed requirements of ice hockey. To increase on-ice speed, the player develops the ability to accelerate as rapidly as possible over short distances from static starts and, more commonly, from rolling starts. Rolling starts are performed in a range of directions: forward, laterally, and to the rear. And the preceding movements occur in a range of distances and speeds that reflect the nature of the game.

Acceleration Speed: On Ice From a Standing Start

Aim   To develop the ability to accelerate over a range of distances.

Action   From a standing start, the athlete skates as rapidly as possible for the chosen distance, typically 5 to 15 meters.

Coaching Points

- Rapidly assume an effective skating acceleration posture.
- Use a driving skating action to accelerate rapidly.

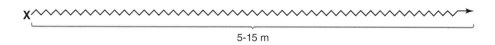

5-15 m

Cruise, Sprint, Cruise

Aim   To develop the ability to accelerate from a rolling start.

Action   The player begins by skating 5 meters at a moderate pace as if cruising in a game situation and then accelerates to a full sprint for 10 meters. Finally, the player decelerates back to the initial pace.

Coaching Points

- Control movements during the buildup.
- Rapidly assume an effective skating acceleration position.
- Use a driving action to accelerate as rapidly as possible.

Variation   The initial movement can take place in a range of directions and speeds to reflect the movement of a player on the ice. The idea is to adjust the body position and accelerate from a range of movement patterns. Additionally, the acceleration can be initiated in response to an external stimulus such as a coach's command.

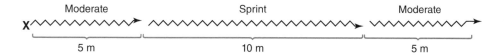

Moderate	Sprint	Moderate
5 m	10 m	5 m

Back and Forward Transition

Aim To develop the ability to accelerate forward after the player has been moving backward.

Action The player skates backward 10 meters, then rapidly stops and accelerates forward for 10 to 15 meters. The player uses a driving acceleration action.

Coaching Points

- Maintain control while skating backward.
- Perform a skating stop.
- Reposition the body into an acceleration posture.
- Skate forward powerfully for the required distance.

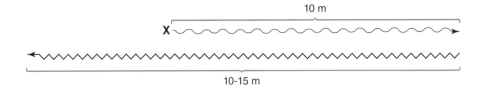

5, 10, 5

Aim To develop the ability to accelerate, stop, and re-accelerate.

Action Three cones are set up 5 meters apart. The player stands next to the center cone then turns to one side and accelerates 5 meters to the end cone. The player turns back the other direction and accelerates 10 meters to the cone at the opposite end. The player turns the other direction and accelerates 5 meters to the center cone. The player repeats the drill, completing the accelerations in the opposite directions.

Coaching Points

- Initiate the movement with a powerful driving action.
- Emphasize appropriate posture.
- Stop rapidly, then accelerate rapidly and powerfully.

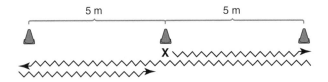

Off-Ice Conditioning

While on-ice conditioning builds the hockey-specific speed capabilities, off-ice conditioning also plays an important role in developing on-ice speed. Off-ice conditioning develops key physical capacities that can translate to more effective on-ice performance. These drills consist of traditional running sprint drills and plyometric-based activities.

Acceleration Running Speed

Aim   To develop the ability to accelerate over a range of short distances.

Action   From a standing start, the athlete accelerates as rapidly as possible for 10 to 20 meters.

Coaching Points

- Maintain an effective acceleration posture with a whole body lean being generated (see chapter 3).
- Emphasize the generation of force through a powerful extension of the rear leg.
- Emphasize a powerful leg drive with the knee of the lead leg being driven forwards and up.
- Utilize a powerful arm action to supplement the drive.

X ———————————————————————————————————————→

10-20 m

Slide Board Sprint

Aim   To develop lateral driving ability together with deceleration mechanics.

Action   The athlete assumes a starting position on the slide board and pushes off explosively in a lateral direction. The athlete decelerates to stop the movement in that direction, using the outside leg, which initially flexes and then rapidly extends to immediately drive off in the opposite direction.

Coaching Points

- Emphasize the leg drive of the outside leg driving the body across the board.
- The arms are held in a bent comfortable position at the side of the body and move rhythmically across the body to support the movement and maintain balance.
- Maintain an athletic posture, with the head in a neutral position, the eyes looking forward, the back flat, and flexion at the ankle, knee, and hip.
- Initiate direction change as rapidly as possible using a cutting action, where the outside leg is flexed and then extended powerfully.

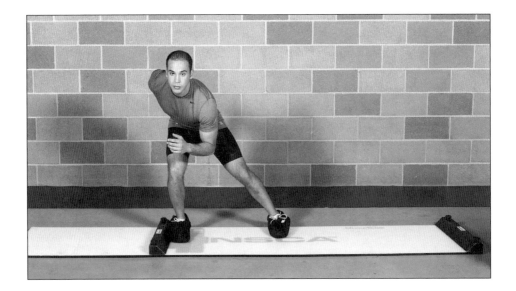

Double-Leg Broad Jump

Aim   To develop explosive strength when moving horizontally.

Action   The athlete assumes a two-footed, square stance and executes a maximum-effort broad jump by pushing off powerfully with both legs (photos *a* and *b*). The athlete lands on the balls of the feet with the thighs no lower than parallel to the ground, with a flat back, and with knees aligned with the feet. The athlete jumps as far as possible without compromising the landing mechanics.

Coaching Points

- Emphasize full extension in the hips during the push-off.
- Use a powerful arm action as shown, with arms driven initially backward and then powerfully forward.
- Land on the balls of the feet (can be a flat-foot if a single jump is performed).
- When landing, keep the thighs parallel to the ground or higher.

Variation   The athlete can progress to performing two or more jumps in a sequence. When performing multiple jumps, the athlete lands on the balls of the feet and tries to spend as little time on the ground as possible to emphasize the stretch-shortening cycle (see chapter 2).

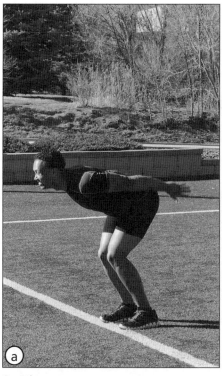

Starting stance.

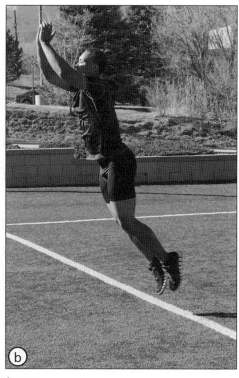

Jump.

Single-Leg Lateral Hurdle Hop

Aim   To develop explosive strength when moving laterally.

Action   The athlete stands on the right leg to the right of a 3-inch (about 7 cm) hurdle. The athlete explosively hops to the left, aiming for maximum distance over the hurdle and lands on the left leg. The athlete holds the landing for a moment before jumping back over the hurdle with the left leg, landing on the right.

Coaching Points

- The jump is initiated with a powerful triple extension of the hip, knee, and ankle of the outside leg.
- Emphasize a powerful arm action.
- The landing is on the ball of the foot, shifting rapidly to the full foot when the athlete holds the position. (When performing repetitions, the landing stays on the balls of the feet.)

Variation   Players can jump off of and land on the same leg. Once players master stability on the landing foot during single hops, they can perform a series of hops in which they change direction immediately upon landing, returning to the start position. When performing a series of hops, emphasis is always on the quality of the movement, so athletes should perform no more than 10 repetitions (5 per leg) in a sequence.

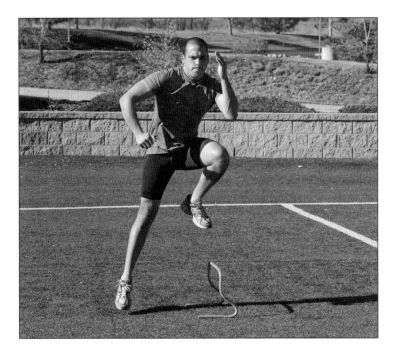

Zigzag Bound

Aim   To develop elastic strength when moving laterally.

Action   A line 10 to 20 meters long is marked on the ground. The athlete stands adjacent to one end of the line, facing the other end. The athlete jumps forward diagonally over the line, initiating the movement with the inside foot and landing on the outside foot. Immediately upon landing, the athlete jumps forward diagonally off the outside foot back over the line, landing on the other foot. The athlete repeats for a specific number of jumps or a specific distance.

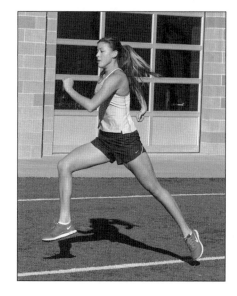

Coaching Points

- Initiate the jump by a powerful triple extension.
- Emphasize a powerful arm action, with both arms initially driven back and then immediately forward.
- Maintain stability by landing on the ball of the foot.

Uphill Running

Aim   To develop explosive strength in triple extension.

Action   The drill takes place on a 20-meter gentle slope of 3 to 6 degrees. The coach or athlete should inspect the surface to make sure there are no hazards such as holes, roots, or large rocks. The athlete accelerates powerfully up the slope for 20 meters and recovers fully by walking slowly back to the start before starting the next repetition.

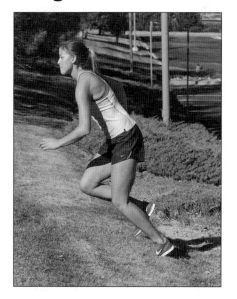

Coaching Points

- Use the acceleration technique outlined in chapter 3.
- Triple extend powerfully with each step, as if pushing the ground away.
- Emphasize a powerful arm action, driving the arms forward to chin level and then powerfully back behind the body.

Sled Pull

Aim   To develop effective driving mechanics and enhance capabilities.

Action   The athlete dons a shoulder harness attached to a sled. Approximately 10 percent of the athlete's bodyweight is added to the sled. The athlete accelerates powerfully from a standing staggered start, continuing for 15 to 20 meters.

Coaching Points

- Attain the acceleration posture described in chapter 3.
- Emphasize a powerful driving action, with full triple extension of the ankle, knee, and hip.
- A powerful arm action complements the driving action of the legs.

RUGBY

Ian Jeffreys

Rugby is one of the most physically demanding sports, requiring high levels of nearly every component of fitness. Of these, speed ranks highly in differentiating between levels of performance and is therefore valued within the game. For this reason, a speed training program needs to be a part of an overall conditioning program for players in all positions and at all levels of performance. The nature of the program will be different depending on the training levels of the athletes, their technical competence, their physical capacity, and also the requirements of the game.

SPEED IN RUGBY

The success of a speed development program is judged on its ability to transfer to, and therefore enhance, onfield performance—the essence of gamespeed. For this reason, a rugby speed development program must start with an analysis of the speed requirements of the sport. The system outlined in chapter 5 provides an ideal mechanism by which to break down rugby speed requirements.

▶ **Typical movement distances.** In term of distances run, differences exist between playing positions and also between off-ball and on-ball requirements. Distances run with the ball are relatively short for all playing positions (less than 10 yards on average) with the average length of run being longer for the outside backs than for the inside backs and for the forwards respectively. Off-ball runs tend to be longer, with the average length being longer for outside backs, inside backs, and forwards, and the back-row forwards typically sprinting greater distances than front-five forwards. Based on this, acceleration plays a greater role in rugby than maximum-speed running for all positions, with the latter playing its greatest role for the outside backs. Acceleration ability needs to be developed from standing starts and from rolling starts of different distances.

▶ **Typical movement directions.** In terms of the directions run, most running is forward but with considerable requirements for direction change. These direction changes are often acute, requiring a cutting step. Others are gentler, requiring a curved pattern. These direction changes are almost entirely perceptually stimulated, with the player reading and reacting to a host of external stimuli, such as the movement of opponents, the movement of the ball, and the movement of teammates. Drills that combine straight-line running with curved running and direction changes are a vital element in a rugby speed development program.

▶ **Typical starting patterns and movement combinations.** Most starts are to the front, from both standing and a rolling motion. Rolling starts are typically linear, although some defensively based sprints may be initiated from a lateral motion. The typical distances of the rolling starts vary by position. For positions close to breakdown situations, rolling starts generally occur over a short distance, often generating forward momentum before a tackle or receiving a ball in attack. For positions away from breakdowns, such as the outside backs, rolling starts are often longer, with the player generating speed before receiving the ball. Exceptions to this occur when forwards provide defensive cover, and in this case, the rolling starts are much longer.

▶ **Perceptual stimuli.** Rugby speed is largely dictated by the ability to respond and move to appropriate perceptual stimuli. Much movement comes after a breakdown situation, and offensively, the movement initially is in response to the ball movement. Defensively, movement is in response to opposition movement together with ball movement. As offensive movement continues, speed requirements are in response to how the game unfolds, and stimuli can be a combination of teammate motion, opposition motion, and ball motion.

▶ **Link to skills.** Offensively, players need to be able to integrate the ball into their execution of speed at some time, whether carrying the ball, catching the ball, or passing the ball. Although most movement occurs off the ball, the ability to carry out these key tasks at speed is important. Defensively, the player needs to be able to make tackles, so must be able to decelerate under control and carry out a tackle at any time. Drills can be developed that incorporate these skills into speed-based activities.

Based on the rugby needs analysis, the following key areas need to be addressed:

▶ Accelerative ability from both static and rolling starts, using rolling starts in a generally linear direction and the distance depending on the playing position

▶ Direction-change ability, both sharp (cutting) and more gentle (curved running)

▶ Maximum-speed ability, predominantly for outside backs

▶ Decelerative ability linked with direction change and sport-skill production

IMPLICATIONS OF SPEED IN RUGBY

Speed is a highly prized asset in rugby and can often differentiate one player from another. Rugby is a collision game, and the generation of momentum is critical to these collisions. Momentum is the product of mass and velocity, so the greater a player's speed capacity, the greater chance that player has of being successful in collision situations.

Speed is a major asset both offensively and defensively. For example, offensive players with greater speed capacities have a greater range of attacking options, allowing them to create and exploit space. Conversely, defensive players lacking speed have an inherent weakness, as they are less able to close down space to make defensive plays. The development of speed should be a key component of any rugby development program.

RUGBY-SPECIFIC DRILLS

Although the following drills improve rugby speed, they should be seen as part of a bigger recipe for success. Speed is dependent on a range of physical abilities, including maximum-force capacity, the rate of force development, and the effectiveness of the stretch-shortening cycle as highlighted in chapter 1. Therefore, coaches and athletes should supplement this work with a strength and power program to maximize its effectiveness. This section provides three types of drills:

▶ Acceleration drills
  • Harness drive (single exchange down and up)
  • Get up and go
  • Linear acceleration dash
  • Linear rolling start
▶ Change-of-direction drills
  • Run and cut
  • Run to daylight
  • Rugby-specific curved running
  • Get past (defender moving forward)
▶ Maximum-speed drill
  • Acceleration run

Harness Drive (Single Exchange Down and Up)

Aim   To develop the ability to drive the knee of the lead leg forward and up, while simultaneously driving the opposite leg down into the ground, holding an acceleration posture.

Action   The athlete stands facing forward with a belt around the waist. The belt is linked to a rope that is held firmly by a partner. This allows the athlete to assume a 45-degree angle. From this posture, the athlete lifts one knee forward and up into a knee-drive position, briefly holding this position. The athlete drives the same leg down into the ground, simultaneously driving the other leg forward and up, again briefly holding this position (photos a and b). The athlete performs this three to five times with each leg. The actions result in forward movement by the athlete.

Coaching Points
- The athlete maintains a straight-line posture with no break at the hip.
- The drive knee moves forward and up with the foot dorsiflexed.
- The exchange of legs should be forceful and rapid without a change in posture.

Variation   This can be developed to double (2 actions, ending up in the same start position) and triple (3 actions) exchanges.

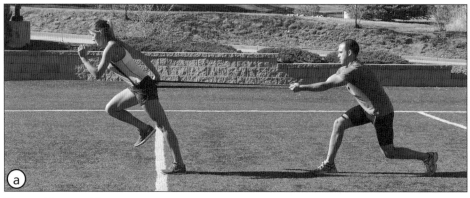

Knee-drive position.

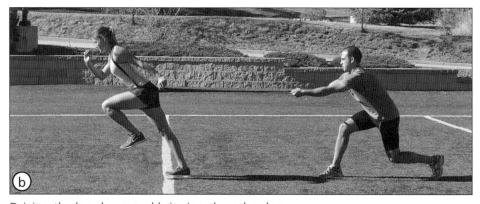

Driving the leg down and bringing the other leg up.

Get Up and Go

Aim   To develop the ability to accelerate from a low body position, which is especially important when accelerating into a potential contact situation.

Action   The athlete lies prone on the ground (photo *a*). On a self-start or a signal from the coach, the athlete lifts out of the start position and sprints forward for a given distance, such as 10 yards (photo *b*).

Coaching Points

- The athlete maintains a straight-line posture, with no break at the hip.
- The athlete maintains a low position throughout the initial acceleration.
- The athlete drives forward and up and should never rise straight up.
- The drive knee moves forward and up, and the foot is dorsiflexed.

Variation   This drill can be performed in competition against other players. Players line up on a start line, and on a signal from the coach sprint for a given distance, such as 10 yards, and try to get to the finish line first.

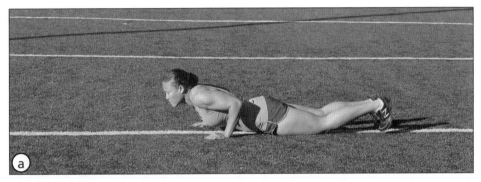

Starting position.

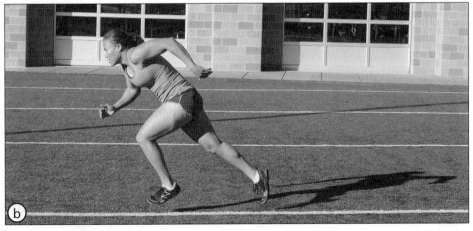

Sprinting.

Linear Acceleration Dash

Aim To develop linear accelerative ability from a standing start.

Action Two cones are placed 10 to 30 yards apart, The distance reflects the requirements of the athlete's playing position. The athlete assumes a defensive position, normally a staggered standing start. On a self-start or signal, the athlete accelerates as quickly as possible for the given distance. The athlete assumes an acceleration posture with the center of mass ahead of the base of support. The athlete focuses on taking powerful, fast strides. The leading knee drives forward and up, and the foot is dorsiflexed through this process.

Coaching Points

- A powerful arm drive through the full range of motion (hip to shoulder) contributes to the ground forces. The arm angle can open slightly on the backward movement to allow more time for force application.
- Foot contact is on the balls of the feet.
- The eyes focus forward not down, enabling the athlete to see the sport action on the field.

Variation Distances can be varied, and athletes can start to the front, to the side, and to the rear. Once athletes have developed the technique, the coach can add competition and use a range of starting mechanisms, such as ball movement.

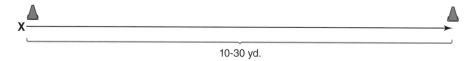

10-30 yd.

Linear Rolling Start

Aim To develop the ability to accelerate from a rolling start.

Action Three cones are placed in a line; the distance between the first two cones is an initial movement zone, and the distance between the second and third cones is an acceleration zone. The athlete moves between the first two cones and on reaching the second cone, accelerates for the given distance. The lengths of the zones reflect typical movement patterns. For example, distances for tight forwards might be 5 yards for initial movement and 5 yards for a sprint. Distances for wingers might be a 15-yard build-up and 15 to 30 yards for the sprint.

Coaching Points

- The athlete maintains control during the initial movement.
- The athlete drives the legs and arms powerfully when accelerating.

Variation The athlete can vary the distance for the initial movement and subsequent movement. The change in pace can be self-directed or triggered by an external signal.

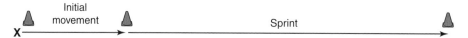

Initial movement

Sprint

Run and Cut

Aim   To develop the ability to change direction through a cut step and then to accelerate.

Action   Two cones are set up 5 yards apart. The athlete assumes an athletic position at cone 1, and then runs toward cone 2, decelerating to make a cut step at the cone. After making the cut step, the athlete immediately accelerates away at approximately 45 degrees. The athlete plants the cutting foot wider than the knee, which is in turn wider than the hips. The drill maximizes the lateral distance the athlete can move and resembles trying to avoid a tackle. Repetitions alternate between cuts to the right and cuts to the left.

Coaching Points

- The foot is planted straight ahead and lands nearly flat, but with weight toward the ball of the foot.
- The body weight stays within the base of support, allowing the athlete to maintain an effective line of force.
- Acceleration should take place immediately after the cut.

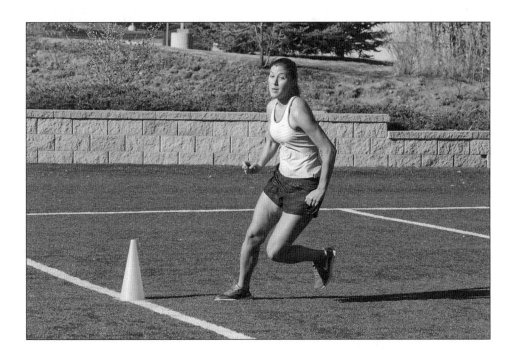

Run to Daylight

Aim   To develop the ability to make a cut step in response to a stimulus and to accelerate from this direction change.

Action   The athlete assumes an athletic position on cone 1, facing cone 2, which is 8 yards away. The coach stands 2 yards behind cone 2. The athlete runs toward cone 2 and decelerates on approaching the cone. As the athlete nears cone 2, the coach makes a lateral move to one side of the cone. The athlete makes a cut step and accelerates in the direction opposite the coach's movement.

Coaching Points

- The cutting foot is planted wider than the knee, which is in turn wider than the hip. The foot is planted straight ahead and almost flat, but with weight toward the ball of the foot.
- The body weight stays within the base of support, allowing the athlete to maintain an effective line of force.
- The athlete accelerates immediately after the cut.

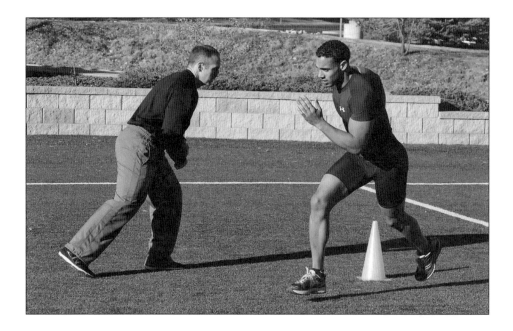

Rugby-Specific Curved Running

Aim   To develop the ability to run in curved patterns and to perfect gentle changes in direction as required during a rugby game.

Action   A series of poles are set up to simulate the curved running patterns found in a rugby game, for example, running at, pinning, and then running around a defender. The athlete sprints through the course, maintaining speed through all of the sections. The athlete leans into the curve. The foot lands under the center of mass, on the balls, and toward the outside of the foot. The recovery leg rapidly cycles, creating a rapid cadence.

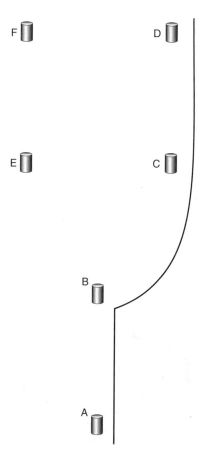

Coaching Points

- The athlete's posture is upright or leaning slightly forward in a straight line.
- The body lean into the curve should be through the whole body
- The arms swing through the full range of motion, with the hands moving from the hip to shoulder level.
- The knee of the lead leg drives forward and up, and the foot is dorsiflexed during this action.

Variation   The coach or athlete can set up a variety of patterns that replicate given tasks in rugby. For example, the coach can set up a pattern that mimics the wide arc movement that a hooker would take on a lineout to receive a pass off the scrum half.

Get Past (Defender Moving Forward)

Aim   To develop the ability to beat a defender and accelerate and to develop the ability to track an opponent's movements forward while maintaining a defensive position.

Action   Two athletes perform the drill, one assuming an offensive role and the other a defensive role. A zone approximately 10 to 20 meters long and 15 to 20 meters wide is marked. The offensive player stands at one end of the marked area at cone 1, which is placed in the middle of that side of the area. The defensive athlete assumes an athletic position at cone 2, at the other end of the zone from the offensive athlete. The offensive athlete moves forward and tries to get to the opposite end of the zone without being tagged by the other athlete. This should require a change of direction followed by a rapid acceleration. The defensive athlete moves forward and adjusts her movements to try to tag the offensive athlete. Athletes should reverse roles on subsequent repetitions.

Coaching Points

- The defender decelerates to a jockeying position and adjusts this in response to the attacker's movements.
- When changing direction, players use the cutting action described in the run and cut drill.
- Athletes accelerate immediately after the cut.

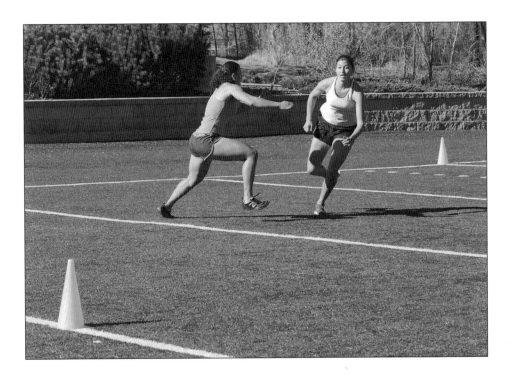

Acceleration Run

Aim   To develop the running action and to learn to change gears at pace.

Action   A series of four cones are set up 20 yards apart. The athlete runs the 60-yard course, increasing running speed in each 20-yard section and attaining maximum speed in the last section. Emphasis is on attaining maximum speed in the last 20 yards and to changing gears in the earlier sections.

Coaching Points

- The athlete's posture is upright or slightly forward, with the body in a straight line.
- The arms swing through a full range of motion, with the hands moving from the hip to shoulder level.
- The knee drives forward and up, and the foot is dorsiflexed during this action. The recovery leg cycles rapidly to create a rapid cadence.
- The foot lands under the center of mass, and on the ball of the foot.

Variation   The distances can be varied to reflect the specific requirements of different positions. The outside backs run the greatest distances.

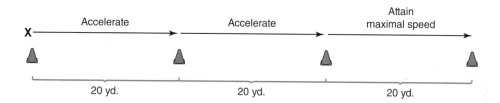

SOCCER

Ian Jeffreys

Speed is a vital component in soccer and plays a key role in determining success in all playing positions. When the goalkeeper sprints off the line to smother the ball at the feet of the oncoming striker or the striker surges to the near post to head home a corner, it's clear that greater speed can significantly enhance the performance of any player.

SPEED IN SOCCER

Part of a speed development program is its ability to transfer to, and thus enhance, on-field performance—the essence of gamespeed. For this reason, a soccer speed development program starts with an analysis of the speed requirements of soccer. The system outlined in chapter 5 provides an ideal mechanism by which to break down soccer speed requirements.

▶ **Typical movement distances.** In terms of the distances run, these are predominantly short, usually 5 to 10 yards (Jeffreys 2007a). In terms of playing positions, distances are shortest for central defenders and goal-keepers, followed successively by strikers, wingers, central midfielders, and wingbacks. Even the longer runs of wingbacks are often a combination of submaximal efforts and much shorter all-out sprints. For this reason, acceleration from standing and especially rolling starts should form a significant part of the speed training of soccer players and should be a key focus for soccer-specific speed development. Developing maximal speed is important for wingers, central midfielders, and wing backs and can also help in speed economy as covered in chapter 2.

▶ **Typical movement directions.** Although accelerative ability is crucial to soccer performance, soccer speed is multidirectional in nature. Seldom is movement in a single direction for an extended period, and motion analysis demonstrates that there are changes in motion every few seconds. Soccer motion involves running linearly, laterally, and to the rear, and running in combinations of these patterns. Therefore, players need to be able to initiate movement in a linear, lateral, and posterior direction. Again, this needs to be developed from static starts and especially from rolling starts. Additionally, there is a frequent requirement to change direction while accelerating. These direction changes can be acute, requiring a sharp cut step, or more gentle in a curved running pattern. The ability to change direction in a variety of ways and subsequent directions is fundamental to soccer speed.

▶ **Typical starting patterns and movement combinations.** Most speed in soccer originates from movement, whether this is a relatively static jockeying position or totally dynamic. While goalkeepers occasionally originate their movements from standing starts, the vast majority of soccer speed originates from a rolling start. Therefore, this should be practiced frequently to maximize the transfer to on-field performance. Rolling starts vary in distance, direction, and preceding movement pattern. For example, rolling starts could involve submaximal running in a range of directions, with the player accelerating in response to an external stimulus. However, this is only a part of the equation because players often undertake a different movement pattern before running: jockeying, side shuffling, backpedaling, backtracking, and so on. Therefore, they need to develop the ability to transition from these movements into accelerative patterns. Here the focus is on the typical combinations seen in soccer and introducing them into the speed training program. Soccer speed sessions should, therefore, include a variety of movement transition patterns and develop the ability to start from a range of initial movement patterns.

▶ **Perceptual stimuli.** Perceptual stimuli play a major role in dictating the movement requirements of soccer. Because soccer players are in relatively constant motion, play includes very few preset movement patterns, and practically all movement is dictated by an external stimulus, normally the movement of the ball, an opponent, or a teammate. The ability to read and react to this type of stimulus is important and emphasizes the role of transition movements in the flow of a game. Players must maintain a position that allows them to read, react to, and move in response to an external stimulus. These types of activities are incorporated into a soccer speed program to maximize the transfer to on-field performance. This type of training should not occur in isolation. The effectiveness of subsequent movement depends on the quality of the movement patterns, and this needs to be developed progressively. Similarly, much of the ability to read the game is developed in soccer-specific sessions. Even in soccer-specific sessions, the quality of the movement patterns should be stressed to ensure that effective motor programs are developed. This requires collaboration with the soccer coach and this will maximize the effectiveness of both the conditioning work and the soccer-specific work.

▶ **Link with sport skills.** The link between speed and sport skills is vital in maximizing gamespeed. Most sprints in soccer end with a soccer-related skill, whether it be offensive (pass, shot, header), or defensive (tackle, header, save). Critical to this is the ability to position the body to be able to carry out this task, and this stresses deceleration ability and transition movements. Drills that combine speed with soccer skills stress the importance of movement patterns and reinforce the work of basic drills that emphasize these movements. In this way, track techniques do not always transfer well into soccer because these techniques do not always place the athlete in a position to carry out soccer-specific skills.

Based on the soccer needs analysis, the following key areas need to be addressed:

▶ Accelerative ability from both static and rolling starts, using rolling starts in a variety of directions and using varied movement patterns

▶ Direction change ability, both sharp (cutting) and gentle (curved running)

▶ Maximum-speed ability for players covering greater distances, such as wingbacks, wingers, and central midfielders

▶ Decelerative ability

IMPLICATIONS OF SPEED IN SOCCER

Enhancing a player's speed can provide significant advantages. These can be applied both offensively and defensively. In simple terms, faster players can get to the ball faster, enabling them to win or maintain possession. This in turn enables their team to dictate play. Additionally, greater speed provides an additional attacking tool because it enables players to go past opponents, which can be a great advantage in an attacking situation. Similarly, greater speed can provide great advantages off the ball. Players with greater speed are better able to create space and accelerate into space, providing a powerful attacking advantage. Defensively, greater speed allows a player to close down space and contain attacking threats.

SOCCER-SPECIFIC DRILLS

Many of the basic speed requirements from the analysis can be developed through the drills in chapter 3. These should form the backbone of a program, The drills outlined here provide a greater degree of soccer specificity. While the drills outlined in this section improve soccer speed, they are part of a bigger recipe for success. Speed is dependent on a range of physical abilities, including maximum force capacity, the rate of force development, and the stretch-shortening cycle ability as highlighted in chapter 1. Therefore, this work needs to be supplemented by a strength-based program to maximize its effectiveness.

▶ Acceleration drills
  • Wall drive (single exchange)
  • Lateral ball drop
  • Multidirectional rolling starts

► Change-of-direction drills
  • Side shuffle and cut
  • Run to space
  • Soccer-specific curved running
  • Get past (defender moving backward)
► Maximum-speed drills
  • Acceleration run
  • Ins and outs
► Deceleration drills
  • Decelerate to a staggered defensive stance
  • Decelerate to a skill

Wall Drive (Single Exchange)

Aim To develop the ability to drive the knee of the lead leg forward and up while holding an acceleration posture.

Action The athlete stands approximately a yard away from a wall and assumes a 45-degree body lean, with the hands against the wall, supporting the body. From this posture, the athlete lifts the right knee forward and up toward the wall and into a knee-drive position, briefly holding this position. The athlete drives the right leg down into the ground, simultaneously driving the left leg forward and up, again briefly holding this position.

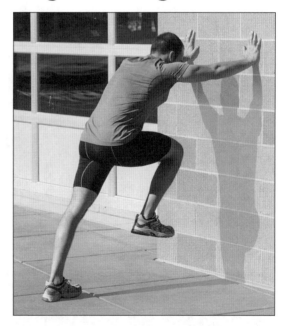

Coaching Points
  • The athlete maintains a straight-line posture with no break at the hip.
  • The drive knee moves forward and up with the foot dorsiflexed.
  • The exchange of legs should be forceful and rapid, but should not result in a change in posture.

Variation This can be developed to double (2 actions, where the athlete returns to the start position) and triple exchanges (3 actions).

Lateral Ball Drop

Aim   To develop the ability to accelerate laterally in reaction to a stimulus.

Action   The athlete assumes a staggered stance, and a coach or partner faces the athlete from a position 5 meters to the side of the athlete. The coach or partner holds a soccer ball in front at shoulder height. The athlete faces forward and looks at the ball by turning only the head (photo *a*). The partner drops the ball and on that signal, the athlete performs a hip turn and accelerates forcefully to reach and control the ball before it bounces a second time (photo *b*). The athlete drives the outside leg forward and then accelerates.

Coaching Points

- The athlete performs a hip turn, opening the hips toward the direction of motion, and shifting the body weight in this direction.
- Strides are as rapid and powerful as possible.

Variation   The distance between the athlete and partner is increased after each successful attempt. The athlete can perform a variety of skills, such as shooting, passing, and initiating a dribble. The partner can drop the ball in front of the athlete or to the rear.

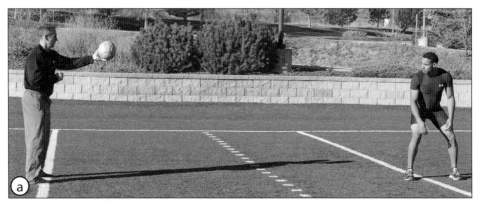

Starting position.

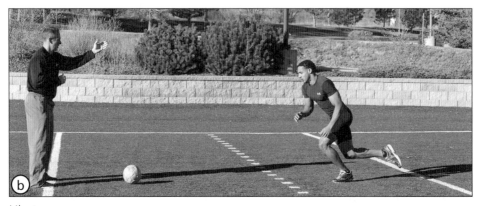

Hip turn.

Multidirectional Rolling Starts

Aim To develop the ability to accelerate from a range of rolling starts.

Action Two cones are placed to mark an initial movement zone, with a further cone placed to represent an acceleration zone. The setup depends on the choice of initial movement and subsequent movement. The athlete moves between the first two cones and on reaching the second cone, accelerates in a given direction for a given distance towards the third cone. Soccer movement is characterised by multiple movement combinations. Therefore, rolling starts can be initiated from a range of directions and into a range of subsequent directions, and the subsequent direction of acceleration (to the side or straight ahead) can vary depending on the aim of the drill.

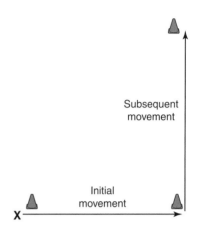

Coaching Points

- The athlete maintains a position of control during the initial movement.
- The athlete drives the legs and arms powerfully when accelerating.

Variation A variety of patterns can be developed by adjusting the initial movement and subsequent movement. The change in pace can be self-directed or initiated by an external signal.

Side Shuffle and Cut

Aim To develop an effective cutting step to change direction.

Action The drill uses two cones set up 5 yards apart. The athlete assumes an athletic position facing one cone, with the other cone to the athlete's side. The athlete side shuffles to the other cone, and at the second cone, performs a cutting action and side shuffles back to the first cone (photos a and b). When cutting, the cutting foot plants wider than the knee, which is in turn wider than the hip. The athlete plants the foot pointed straight ahead and nearly flat, with weight toward the ball of the foot to allow a greater force to be applied. The athlete pushes aggressively with this foot to side shuffle back in the opposite direction.

Coaching Points

- During the side shuffle, the body weight stays within the base of support, allowing the athlete to maintain an effective line of force.
- The foot does not flair out when planted. It stays pointing straight ahead.

Variation The athlete can perform the drill as a single repetition or as a series of repetitions, ensuring that an equal number of cuts are performed on each leg during the practice. Once the athlete masters the original drill, change of direction can be initiated on an external signal.

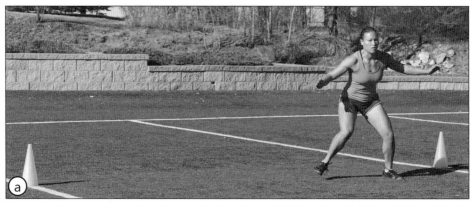

Side shuffle.

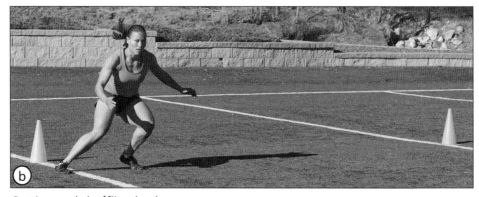

Cutting and shuffling back.

Run to Space

Aim   To develop the ability to accelerate to a given point in a soccer-specific context.

Action   A 10-meter-square is marked with cones at each corner. Two athletes stand facing each other within the square. One assumes an offensive role and the other a defensive role. The offensive player's aim is to create space and accelerate to a cone, while the defensive player aims to maintain the initial distance between them and if possible prevent the offensive athlete from getting to the cone or getting to the cone first. The offensive athlete moves first, trying to manipulate the defender in order create space and subsequently accelerate to one of the four cones (photos *a* and *b*). The drill ends after 3 seconds or whenever the athlete reaches the cone. Athletes reverse roles on subsequent repetitions.

Coaching Points

- Both athletes maintain jockeying positions before the movement.
- The athlete accelerates as described in chapter 3.

Variation   This drill can be varied by changing the area covered or the position the athlete tries to get to (this may be random or predetermined by the coach) or by adding a skill requirement such as receiving a pass on reaching the cone.

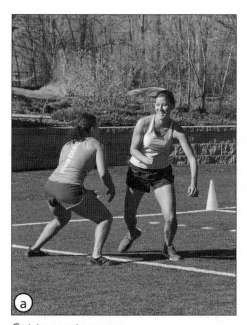

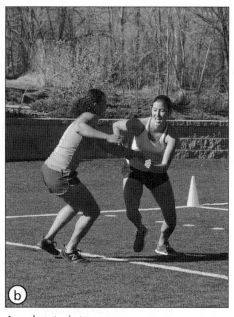

Cut to create space.

Accelerate into space.

Soccer-Specific Curved Running

Aim   To develop the ability to run in curved patterns and to perfect gentle changes in direction.

Action   A series of poles are placed in a pattern simulating the curved running typical of soccer. For example, the drill can replicate the pattern center forwards may run in creating space as they move toward the near post to receive a cross. The athlete sprints through the course, maintaining speed through all the sections. Throughout the pattern, the athlete's posture is tall but leaning into the curve with the lean being a whole body lean.

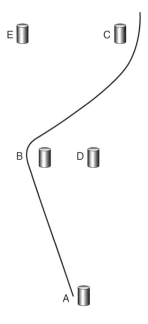

Coaching Points

- The arm swings through a full range of motion, with the hands moving from the hip to shoulder level.

- Any lean should be initiated through the whole body, and with the athlete still running tall.

- The knee drives forward and up, and the foot on that leg is dorsiflexed during this action. The recovery leg cycles through rapidly to create a quick cadence.

- The foot lands under the center of mass and on the ball of the foot a little toward the outside as the athlete leans into the curve.

Variation   A variety of patterns can be set up to replicate different tasks in soccer, such as a wing back running an arc outside a full back or a central midfielder running a curve away from a defender.

Get Past (Defender Moving Backward)

Aim   To develop the offensive ability to beat a defender and accelerate and to develop the defensive ability to track an opponent's movements while moving backward and then to accelerate.

Action   Two athletes perform the drill, one assuming an offensive role and the other a defensive role. A zone approximately 15 yards wide and 20 yards long is a marked, although the size can vary depending on the specific aim of the exercise. For example, smaller areas stress the need to create space in a tight area. The offensive player stands at one end of the marked area at cone 1, which is placed in the middle of that side of the area. The defensive athlete assumes an athletic position at cone 2, which is placed 2 yards in front of the offensive athlete. The drill starts on the first movement of the offensive athlete, who moves forward trying to get to the end of the zone by making a rapid acceleration at some point in the drill. The defensive athlete initially backpedals and then adjusts between movements, tracking the offensive athlete's movements, attempting to stay close to the offensive player through the drill. The player accelerates in response to the attacker's movement. Athletes reverse roles on subsequent repetitions.

Coaching Points

- Effective postures are maintained during the initial movements. For the defensive athlete this requires an athletic position while backtracking. For the offensive player this requires an adjustment between a running pattern and a deceleration pattern to enable an effective cut to take place.
- Direction changes are performed with a cutting action, and athletes accelerate using proper form.

Variation   Variations can be introduced, including changes in distances, changes in directions, different instructions to the players, and the addition of skills, such as reacting to the ball.

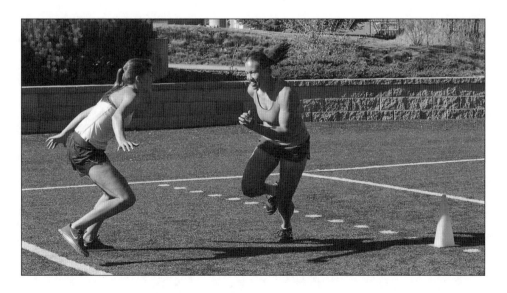

Acceleration Run

Aim   To develop a maximum-speed running action and the ability to change gears at pace.

Action   A series of cones 20 yards apart create a 60-yard course. The athlete runs the course, increasing speed in each 20-yard section so that maximum speed is attained in the last section. The goal is to attain maximum speed in the last 20-yards by changing gears effectively in the earlier sections. During the pattern, the athlete's posture is upright or leaning slightly forward in a straight line.

Coaching Points

- The arm swings through a full range of motion, with the hands moving from the hip to shoulder level.
- The knee of the lead leg drives forward and up, and the foot is dorsiflexed during this action. The recovery leg cycles through rapidly to create a quick cadence.
- The foot lands under the center of mass and on the ball of the foot.

Variation   The distances can be varied.

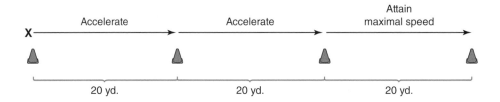

Ins and Outs

Aim   To develop the ability to relax at speed.

Action   Five cones are placed 15 yards apart. The athlete runs the 60-yard course increasing running speed in each 15-yard section so that the athlete attains maximum speed in the second to last 15-yard section. In the final section, the athlete maintains speed while remaining relaxed, pulling back the effort to 90 to 95 percent.

Coaching Points

- The athlete's posture is upright or leaning slightly forward in a straight line.
- The arm swings through a full range of motion, with the hands moving from the hip to shoulder level.
- Remind the athlete to relax.
- The knee of the lead leg drives forward and up, and the foot is dorsiflexed during this action.
- The foot lands under the center of mass and on the ball of the foot.
- The recovery leg cycles through rapidly, creating a quick cadence.

Variation   The out phase of the drill can occur earlier in the sequence, with the athlete returning to maximum speed for a subsequent section.

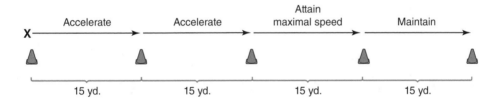

Decelerate to a Staggered Defensive Stance

Aim   To develop the ability to decelerate into a staggered defensive stance.

Action   The athlete assumes an athletic position at cone 1, facing a second cone placed 5 yards away. The athlete runs forward toward cone 2 and decelerates on approaching the cone by lowering the center of mass and shortening the stride (photo a). At the cone, the athlete assumes a staggered athletic position with either foot leading (photo b). This replicates a defensive position, where a defender tries to channel the offensive player in a given direction.

Coaching Points

- The feet are wider apart in an athletic position (hip width or slightly wider) and bodyweight is over the balls of the feet.
- In a staggered athletic stance, one foot is slightly in front of the other, resulting in the body facing toward the left or right.

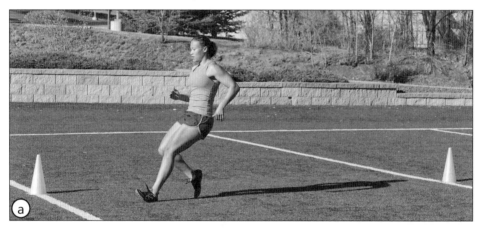

Athlete decelerates.

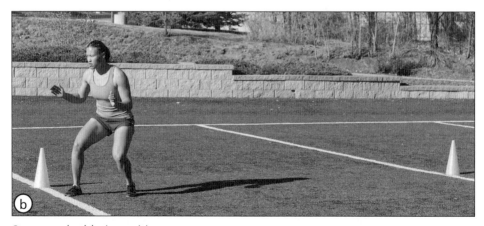

Staggered athletic position.

Decelerate to a Skill

Aim To develop the ability to decelerate and carry out a soccer skill.

Action The athlete assumes an athletic position at cone 1. Cone 2 is 5 to 10 yards ahead. A coach or partner stands with a soccer ball near cone 2. The athlete runs toward cone 2 and then decelerates to be able to carry out a soccer skill (e.g., making a shot, controlling a pass ball, making a save). As the athlete decelerates, the coach or partner feeds the ball in a manner appropriate to the desired skill, and the athlete performs the skill (photos *a* and *b*). This skill can be predetermined or the athlete can be given options and asked to respond according to what evolves as the ball is delivered.

Coaching Points

- The athlete lowers the center of mass while decelerating and rapidly adjusts the stance in preparation for the skill.
- The athlete shortens the stride length as he or she approaches the cone.
- The feet are placed wider apart (hip width or slightly wider) to assume an athletic position, and the bodyweight is over the balls of the feet.

Variation Variations can be made in the distances used, the initial speeds of movement, and the skill performed.

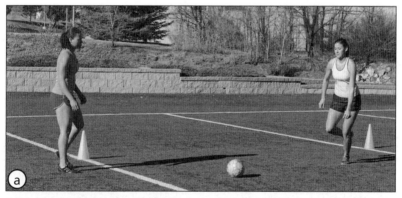

Athlete accelerates to the ball.

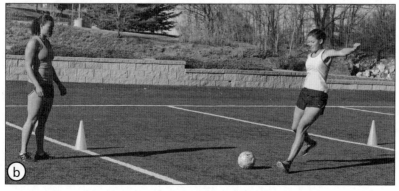

Athlete decelerates to shoot the ball.

TENNIS

Diane Vives

Tennis is a multidirectional sport consisting of short sprints, rapid changes of direction, and intermittent short recovery periods, all interspersed with tennis-specific skills. The specific movements vary from point to point and are dictated by the requirements of the game. The sprints are determined by anticipating the opponent's next action as well as the subsequent flight and speed of the ball. Because this creates context-specific speed requirement, this section focuses on developing sport-specific speed for the tennis player.

SPEED IN TENNIS

Given the specificity of tennis speed, it is vital to evaluate the movement demands of competitive tennis matches. In a typical game the points usually last less than 10 seconds with 20 to 25 seconds between points (Kovacs 2009). Although these times can vary depending on the surface the game is played on.

During a point, the tennis player averages four changes of direction. However, this can range from 1 to 15 changes of direction depending on the length of the point and the type of surface (Kovacs 2009). Studies have shown that during match play, 80 percent of strokes require movements that are 2.5 meters or less in distance, compared to just 5 percent of distances that are more than 4.5 meters between strokes (Kovacs 2004 and 2009, Roetert et al. 2005). Maximum distances covered are typically between 8 and 12 meters. This emphasizes the need for speed over short distances. We can therefore conclude that power, power endurance (the ability to sustain high levels of power over extended exertions), and speed are the predominant physical components of the game and therefore need to be the focus of conditioning programs for tennis.

In evaluating the movements common to tennis, we see sprints forward to the net (less than 20 percent), sprints back to the baseline (less than 8 percent), sprints laterally to cover the width of the court (more than 70 percent), and a combination of those that runs in a diagonal direction to cover the shortest distance to the ball. Of these directions of movement, recent studies show that more than 70 percent of movement in tennis is side to side (Kovacs 2009). This fact supports the relevance of lateral speed training in order to enhance tennis-specific speed on the court.

Another important aspect of tennis speed, given the short distances involved, is the use of specific strategies for first-step quickness and starts for acceleration. Movement depends on the opponent's actions, and a player needs to assume starting positions that allow for subsequent movement in multiple directions. A technique to enable rapid first steps is the split step, which prepares the athlete for forward or lateral acceleration. In recent years this strategy to break inertia and produce a powerful first step has gone through an evolution in higher levels of play (Roetert and Ellenbecker 2001). Because of advances in the speed of the sport and the coach's ability to use video analysis, the split step has evolved. Instead of landing simultaneously and parallel, elite players use the modern split step in which the player reacts in the air during the split and lands with the foot farthest from the ball a split second before the opposite foot (Roetert and Ellenbecker 2001). In lateral movement, the athlete is faster using a split step (Kovacs 2009, Matsuda et al. 2005),

Other strategies for quick starts include the pivot step and the gravity step, which are used for lateral acceleration. The pivot step involves pivoting on the lead foot while turning the hips toward the ball and making the first step toward the ball with the opposite leg (Kovacs 2009). The gravity step, on the other hand, engages the first step by bringing the lead foot toward the body and away from the intended direction similar to how a drop step is used in forward movement. This step toward the body shifts the center of gravity to the edge of or just outside the base of support and angles the body for force production in the intended direction. Although both of these strategies work for lateral acceleration, researchers and many coaches suggest the gravity step is faster than the pivot step when a player needs to move laterally on the tennis court (Kovacs 2009).

IMPLICATIONS OF SPEED IN TENNIS

Having looked at the dominant factors that positively affect tennis-specific speed, it is possible to identify components that the strength coach or trainer can use to enhance a tennis player's speed on the court. Tennis is a combination of stops, starts, changes of direction, and short sprints. It is important to understand the key components that will translate into better speed and changes of direction on the tennis court, and understanding these components will make the use of the drills in the following section more effective.

To be successful, an athlete must exhibit dynamic balance. This is the ability to keep the center of gravity over the base of support while moving. Optimal control of dynamic balance allows for proper force production in any direction. If the athlete is out of balance and the center of gravity is outside the base of support, the athlete cannot be effective, and many times this will increase the ground contact time or minimize force application. This can result in slower changes of direction and the need to take unnecessary recovery steps, which are counterproductive in tennis.

Another vital component, but one that is often overlooked, is deceleration. Kovacs dubbed deceleration "the forgotten factor in tennis-specific training" (2008). The tennis player's ability to decelerate properly determines how effective the athlete can load and prepare for a movement, how powerfully the movement is expressed, and then how safely the movement is decelerated. Effective deceleration for the lower body lowers the center of gravity, which loads the larger muscles of the lower body, while the center of gravity stays within the base of support. The importance of deceleration training not only applies to speed and performance, but it is also recognized as a factor in reducing the incidence of injury. It has been established that a large number of injuries occur during the deceleration phase of movement, and therefore, effective deceleration training can decrease the likelihood of injury (Kovacs 2008).

To maximize the benefit of these drills it is important to first use closed-skill drills, where the athlete performs a set movement pattern in an unchanging environment. This allows the athlete to develop and stabilize key movement patterns before focusing on more complex, reactive drills. For tennis, reactive training covers movements specific to tennis play on the court and the skills needed to improve performance. This allows the athlete to put skills and movement patterns together in a predictable setting to optimize development of coordination and specific training components. Once the athlete has mastered the closed-skill drills these can be progressed to open-skill drills in which unpredictable stimuli, such as a tennis ball toss, a coach's verbal cue, or a gesture with the racket are added. This allows the coach to provide a gamelike atmosphere in training while knowing that time is being invested in skills that will translate to the tennis court.

Although the basic skills and mechanics of linear acceleration are not dominant movements in tennis, training these skills is beneficial when developing an athlete. Training in forward sprinting can benefit the foundational mechanics for multidirectional speed. Therefore, many of the drills highlighted in chapter 3 can be used in a tennis speed program.

TENNIS-SPECIFIC DRILLS

This section focuses on drills that enhance speed as it relates to tennis. Four types of drills are presented: deceleration, acceleration, change of direction, and reactive open skills. These movement patterns reflect the way speed is applied in a tennis context. These are just examples, so coaches and athletes can add or alternate drills that address these basic abilities.

- ▶ Deceleration drills
  - Drop squat
  - One-leg balance to split landing
  - Skater for stability

▶ Acceleration drills
- Lateral skip
- Speed shift with split step
- Hurdle jump

▶ Change-of-direction drills
- Slide board sprint
- Tennis shuttle run
- X-pattern
- Z-pattern cut

▶ Reactive open-skill drills
- Reactive T
- Competitive fire feet to sprint
- Medicine ball toss and sprint

Progression of drills is an important element of speed development. The drills presented in this section have been constructed to follow a general progression that both reduces the chance of injury and maximizes the development of tennis-specific speed. The progressions are as follows:

▶ Slow and stable to fast and explosive
▶ Simple to complex
▶ Single direction to multidirectional
▶ Closed skill to open skill
▶ Body weight to external resistance

Drop Squat

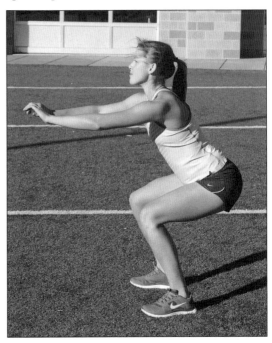

Aim To train the ability to drop the center of mass quickly and under control. This emphasizes the eccentric strength of loading the lower body in a two-foot stance while maintaining proper position and dynamic balance.

Action The athlete starts with the feet hip-width apart in an upright position. The athlete drops the hips back quickly into a squat position, finishing with the thighs just above parallel to the ground and with the feet in a shoulder-width stance. The athlete comes to a complete stop, showing balance and control, before returning to an upright position for the next repetition.

Coaching Points

- The movement emphasizes the hips dropping back. Being too upright and exaggerating the knee bend in the associated movement forward places anterior stress on the knees.
- The eyes are forward, the chest up, and the feet facing forward (not rotated outward).
- The drop is as fast as the athlete can control and the finish is in a balanced and stable position.

Variation Use a partner's hands for resistance on the shoulders to produce a slight overload to the movement. Progress to band resistance at the hips with a 45-degree angle to an anchor on the ground. Light resistance is sufficient to create a significant load. For advanced athletes, the drop squat can be done on a single leg while maintaining strict ankle, knee, and hip alignment.

One-Leg Balance to Split Landing

Aim   To train the strength and position needed to decelerate from both forward and lateral movement. To be successful, the athlete must drop the center of mass and engage the muscles to quickly decelerate while avoiding unwanted extra steps or upper-body movements.

Action   The athlete starts in a single-leg stance with the opposite knee raised to hip level (photo *a*). The athlete initiates the drop by leaning forward. The landing results in a split stance at hip-width apart, with the forward leg's thigh just above parallel to the ground and the torso upright (photo *b*). The opposite arm is forward to execute upper-body counterbalance. The athlete makes a definite pause and demonstrates complete stability at the finish. The athlete repeats on the opposite side.

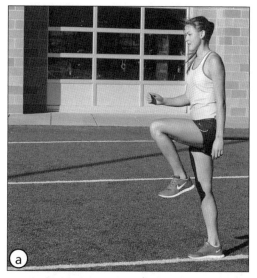

Starting position.

Coaching Points

- Watch for good ankle, knee, and hip alignment on both legs.
- The knee does not collapse outward.
- The landing should be quiet and controlled, and the finish is in a balanced and stable position.
- The side view shows the forward leg in an athletic stance, or power position, at the finish.

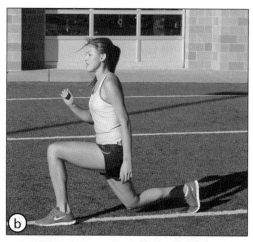

Split step.

Variation   A partner can stand behind the athlete and give a light push at the start of the forward lean to add momentum and overload the landing position. A partner can toss a medicine ball in the direction of the movement for the athlete to catch as she lands. This adds a load to the deceleration position and challenges dynamic stability. Next, the athlete can follow the landing with an immediate explosive push-off back up into the single-leg stance.

The drill can also be completed as a lateral movement by using the same single-leg stance and then leaning directly to the side of the raised leg. That foot lands pointing forward, while ankle, knee, and hip finish in alignment in the power position on that side of the body.

Skater for Stability

Aim   To train the strength and stability needed for powerful change of direction. The goal is to work from a controlled stable landing with a pause to display proper position and balance.

Action   The athlete starts in a single-leg stance and bounds onto the opposite leg in a directly lateral position, landing in a single-leg power position (photos *a* and *b*). The body is not too upright. The athlete pauses in the final position with no movement to demonstrate stability and control. The athlete can start with narrow bounds and progress to wider bounds. A countermovement may be used to initiate the lateral bound if it is quick and crisp with no delay before takeoff.

Coaching Points

- The body's center of gravity and shoulders are over the base of support at landing.
- The feet face forward and do not rotate outward.
- The drill focuses on the stability of the landing position rather than reducing ground contact time and explosiveness.

Variation   The athlete can progress to a diagonal skater by bounding forward and laterally in a zigzag pattern.

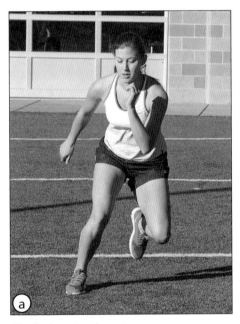 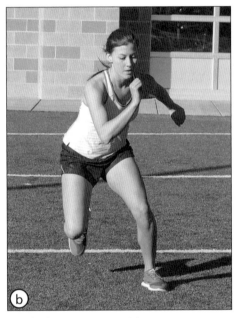

Single-leg starting stance.   Single-leg power position.

Lateral Skip

Aim   To develop lateral acceleration and powerful lateral takeoffs.

Action   The athlete begins by skipping in place and then uses the left leg to force-fully push off using triple extension (of the ankle, knee, hip) to propel the body to the right, or the right leg to propel to the left. The athlete maintains the skipping foot pattern, keeps the shoulders facing forward, and uses consistent contralateral arm motions as in regular skipping.

Coaching Points

- The feet do not cross.
- The athlete drives off the trail leg at an acceleration angle with full extension of the ankle, knee, and hip.

Variation   Resistance can be added by looping a resistance band around the athlete's waist. A partner anchors the band on the ground at a 45-degree angle later-ally from the trail leg. The athlete can combine forward skipping and lateral skipping sequences. External resistance can be applied through a weighted vest. The weight should be no more than 5 to 10 percent of the athlete's body weight.

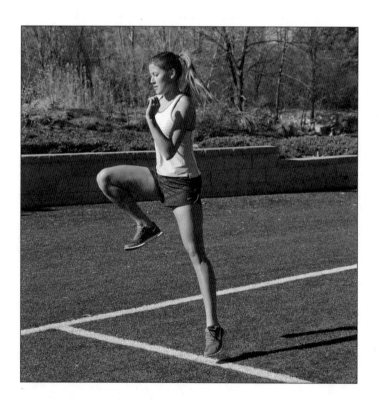

Speed Shift With Split Step

Aim   To develop the ability to accelerate into a sprint from a slower forward movement. Forward acceleration is the emphasis.

Action   Four to six cones are placed 5 yards apart in a straight line. The athlete starts with a slow jog. On reaching the second cone, the athlete uses a split step to initiate a powerful takeoff in a sprint and sprints at full speed to the next cone. At the next cone, the athlete decelerates as quickly as possible into a slow jog. The athlete repeats this pattern until reaching the last cone.

Coaching Points

- Athletes may use either the standard version of the split step or the modern split step, depending on their experience and level of play.
- The athlete drops the center of gravity during deceleration and uses proper mechanics.
- While sprinting, the athlete drives the arm forward and up to shoulder level and pulls the arm back so the hand is at the hip.

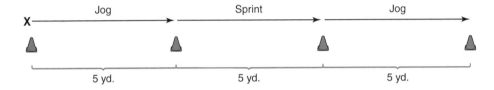

Hurdle Jump

Aim   To improve the athlete's strength and power for acceleration.

Action   Five hurdles are placed approximately 2 feet (about 60 cm) apart. The hurdles are 2 to 18 inches (about 5-45 cm) high depending on the athlete's training history, experience, and progression. The coach approaches the initial height and progression conservatively for beginners. From a shoulder-width stance, the athlete jumps over the hurdles, maintaining a continuous jumping pattern over the series of hurdles. Athletes focus on keeping the feet quiet and jumping over the hurdles in a consistent rhythm. As athletes becomes more experienced, they focus on spending as little time on the ground as possible, as if landing on hot coals. The athlete initially jumps with both feet, then progresses to a single-leg hop.

Coaching Points

- Use no more than five hurdles to ensure the athlete reaches full amplitude on each jump. Limiting the number of hurdles negates the effects of fatigue.
- The progression to higher hurdles should occur in small increments to gradually increase the amplitude and intensity of the jumps.

Variation   After mastering forward jumps, the athlete can also incorporate lateral jumps. The athlete uses proper jumping mechanics.

After athletes master forward and lateral jumps (this could take several weeks), they can perform single-leg hops over the hurdles. The progression starts with single-leg forward hops over lower hurdles and progresses to single-leg lateral hops (lead with both the inside edge of the foot and the outside edge of the foot). Again, the progression to higher hurdles is incremental.

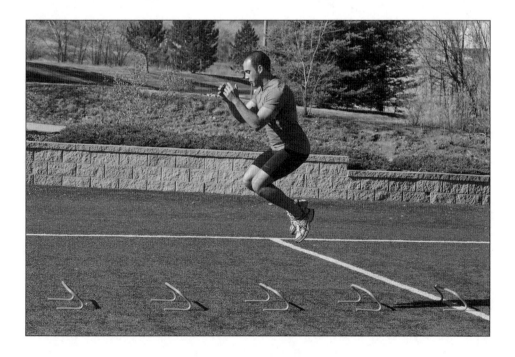

Slide Board Sprint

Aim   To train lateral changes of direction and improve dynamic balance.

Action   The coach chooses a slide board length that allows a proper takeoff and a slide distance that puts the athlete firmly against the opposite side block. This allows proper contact for the repetitions that follow. The athlete starts with one foot against the block, with the upper body rotated toward that foot to "load" the position (photo *a*). The athlete performs four to eight slides as fast as possible (photo *b*). This is intended to be a sprint using explosive, fast repetitions of the slide movement. The athlete focuses on the fast, lateral changes of direction, spending as little time on the blocks as possible. The athlete should use the upper body, arms, and shoulders to assist in loading the push-off, while the torso should remain stable in an athletic position throughout. The arms drive across the body in the direction of travel. The upper body plays a large role in producing a forceful lateral motion.

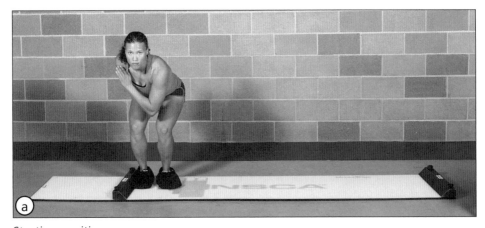

Starting position.

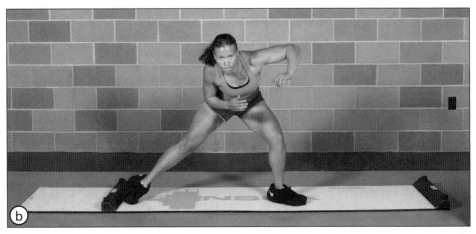

Sliding.

Coaching Points

- The athlete stays in an athletic stance at all times.
- When sliding, the feet are shoulder-width apart.

Variation Advanced athletes can emphasize the push-off by attaching a light band to the waist and anchoring it to the side they are focusing on. The motion is an explosive, resisted push-off and an easy controlled return into position. The athlete repeats on the opposite side. The athlete can add a free weight, which is easy to hold with one hand. The athlete holds the weight in the front hand, thus loading the landing and push-off position, then changes hands midslide to load the opposite side.

Tennis Shuttle Run

Aim To train lateral changes of direction, improve the mechanics of changing direction, and improve the strength and power needed for faster reaction and lateral starts.

Action Three cones are set 5 yards apart in a straight line. The athlete starts at the center cone, parallel with the line of the cones and the right foot in line with the center cone. The athlete sprints to the right side cone and touches it with the right hand. The athlete turns and sprints to the far cone and touches it with the left hand, then turns and sprints back to the center cone.

Coaching Points

- Coach the athlete to lower the center of gravity and decelerate quickly to load the body for the change of direction.
- Use a variety of steps such as the split step, gravity step, or the pivot step to start the drill.
- Dynamic balance is crucial to changing direction as quickly as possible.

Variation To emphasize deceleration and control, two tennis balls can be introduced. The athlete starts with one ball in the hand and the second ball on the left cone. The athlete sprints to the right to first cone and places the ball on it. The athlete sprints to the far left cone, picks up the ball from the top of the cone, and then sprints to the finish. The athlete may use cones of different heights to emphasize different body positions during the direction change, making this drill more tennis specific.

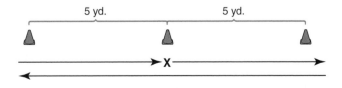

X-Pattern

Aim   To improve multidirectional sprints and the footwork associated with changing directions.

Action   Four cones are placed in a square with sides 5 yards long. The athlete starts at cone 1 and sprints straight ahead to cone 2. The athlete touches cone 2, turns to the right, and then sprints to cone 4. The athlete touches cone 4, turns to the left, and sprints straight ahead to cone 3. The athlete touches cones 3, turns to the left, and then sprints through cone 1. Touching the cones forces a full deceleration and controlled stop so that the athlete must use a powerful start to sprint to the next cone.

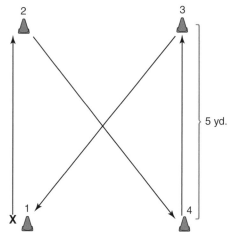

Coaching Points

- The athlete needs to lower the center of mass and shorten their stride length as they decelerate.
- Subsequent acceleration should involve a powerful triple extension at the rear leg, and a powerful drive forward and up with the lead leg.
- Arms should be used powerfully to complement the leg action.

Variation   Athletes may use a combination of skills, such as shuffles and backpedaling mixed with the sprints. The athlete can also perform the drill while a coach or trainer stands at the top of the square in front of cone 1. The athlete sprints in the same pattern as in the original drill, but at cone 1 the coach tosses the athlete a light medicine ball, and the athlete returns it with a rotational toss. The athlete continues to cone 2, and sprints to cone 3, performs a second rotational toss, and then sprints to cone 4.

Z-Pattern Cut

Aim   To develop sharp, crisp cutting skills that improve change-of-direction abilities.

Action   Four cones are set up 5 yards apart in a Z pattern. The athlete starts in a parallel stance at the first cone and sprints diagonally to the next cone and plants the outside foot and sprints to the next cone diagonally and cuts using the outside foot to continue to the last cone. This creates a Z-pattern run. Once the athlete is familiar with the pattern and can execute the cutting movements, the athlete performs the drill at full speed while maintaining proper form and control.

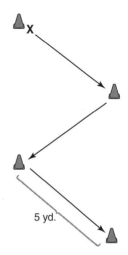

Coaching Points

- Make sure athletes drop their center of gravity as they perform the cutting movement. Do not let the athlete stay upright.
- Coach the athlete to keep the shoulders within the base of support when cutting.

Variation   A weighted vest can load the body and enhance the elastic strength needed for quick changes of direction. The athlete can touch the cone with the hand to emphasize deceleration and starts. The athlete can shuffle to the right and sprint to the left.

Reactive T

Aim   To improve the speed of reaction time and change of direction.

Action   Four cones are set up to create a T pattern. The typical distance between cones 1 and 2 is 10 yards and between cones 3 and 4 is 10 yards, although the distance can be shortened. The athlete starts in an athletic position at cone 1. On the coach's command, the athlete sprints toward cone 2. As the athlete approaches, the coach provides a second command indicating the direction the athlete must cut and go when reaching the middle cone. The athlete next sprints and touches that cone, changes direction, and sprints to the opposite side cone and back to the middle cone and then backpedals to the finish at cone 1.

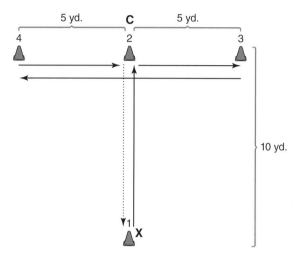

Coaching Points

- The forward sprint should be as fast as possible while maintaining form.
- Give athletes a second command at the midpoint of the sprint to allow them to execute the cut at full speed.
- Coach proper deceleration and starts during the changes of direction.

Variation   Verbal cueing can become more complex by using colors or words for the directions and start. Coaches can introduce visual cues, such as a tennis ball or racket or simply a gesture with the arms.

Competitive Fire Feet to Sprint

Aim   To improve reaction time and improve the strength and power needed for changes of direction.

Action   Four cones are set up to create a box. A fifth cone sits in the center of the square. Each side of the square is 10 yards long. Two athletes start on either side of the cone in the center of the square (photo *a*). On the coach's command both athletes begin quick "fire feet" movements in place. When the coach gives the command of up, middle, or back, both athletes sprint either laterally or diagonally to the designated cone on their side of the square (photo *b*). The athletes touch the cone, change direction, and race the opponent back to the starting position and immediately resume the "fire feet" movements. This is repeated four to six times to complete the drill. Athletes stay on their side of the square and do not cross the middle cone.

Coaching Points

- Use clear verbal or visual cues.
- Encourage the use of good form on changes of direction and a full-speed sprint to and from the cones.

Variation   More complex cues can be used for target cones. The athlete can begin the spring with a split step. The athlete can use different skills, such as skips or shuffles.

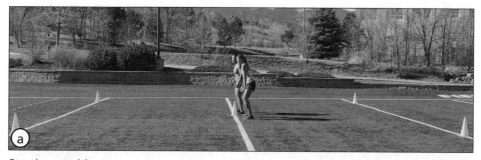

Starting positions.

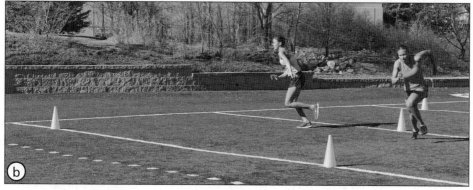

Racing to touch cone.

Medicine Ball Toss and Sprint

Aim   To incorporate a more sport-specific skill while training reaction and speed.

Action   The athlete starts at the center of a baseline within a designated area that mimics the size of the court. Using a light medicine ball, the coach tosses the ball 5 to 15 yards in any direction within the area. The athlete sprints to the ball, letting the ball bounce only once, and then catches and side tosses the ball back to the coach. The toss action should be similar to a forehand or backhand action. At that point the athlete sprints back to the starting location. This is repeated for five tosses. The coach should change the distances and direction of the toss to remain as unpredictable as possible.

Coaching Points

- The athlete should use proper body position and correctly set up for the side toss.
- The athlete should return the ball directly to the coach each time.

Variation   The coach can use commands to designate different tosses, such as overhead toss, chest pass, or scoop. The coach can work with multiple athletes all standing on the baseline. The athletes perform the drill when their name, color, or number is called.

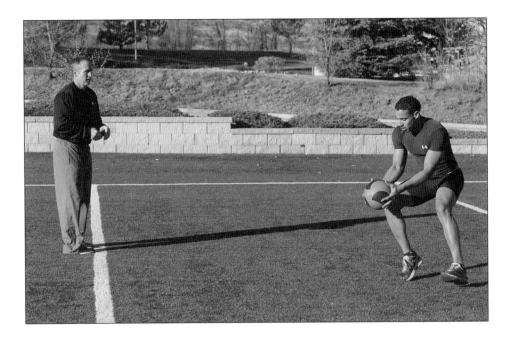

TRACK

Jeremy Sheppard

Nowhere is linear speed as crucial as in the sprint events in track and field, where the men's Olympic 100-meter champion is hailed the fastest man in the world. In essence, the majority of the drills used in chapter 3 along with much of the technical information from chapter 2 has emanated from track sprinting. Therefore, all of the drills outlined in chapter 3 can be applied to the training of track sprinters. However, while speed is crucial in track sprints, previous chapters have highlighted the various components of linear speed, all of which must be addressed in maximizing track sprinting performance.

SPEED IN TRACK

Unlike the other sports, where speed is used in varying contexts and in reaction to an evolving game, track sprinting is predominantly consistent every time. The environment—the running track—is standardized, and the task is predetermined by the event, such as 60 meters on an indoor track or 100 meters on an outdoor track. Tasks are essentially the same for every sprint, with a block start followed by a sequence of on your marks and get start, and then a gun shot. The only variable is temporal pattern of the commands. Since the given task is predetermined, models for sprint technique have far less variability and thus have been far more extensively researched than models for team and court sports.

IMPLICATIONS OF SPEED IN TRACK

It is useful to view track sprinting in five key stages: reaction, acceleration, maximum speed, speed maintenance, and deceleration. The reaction stage constitutes the set position, the reaction to the gun, and the first force production. Each of the remaining stages is determined by the rate of change in velocity (acceleration) and the velocity at which the athlete is sprinting. The acceleration phase encompasses the entire distance in which the athlete is increasing speed from the start; the maximum-speed phase encompasses the distance in which the athlete is at the highest velocity, and the speed maintenance phase is everything thereafter, wherein the athlete maintains maximal velocity. In reality, this last phase may entail a degree of deceleration, depending on the athlete's capacity to maintain maximal speed.

The success of the reaction phase is determined by the speed of reaction to the gun and the subsequent force exerted against the blocks. Ideally, the athlete exerts as great a force as possible in the shortest time possible. After leaving the blocks, the athlete enters the acceleration phase of the sprint, which can be further divided into initial acceleration and transition acceleration. The entire phase is characterized by increasing stride lengths at each distance and shorter ground contact times with distance.

Stride rates also increase. Men typically achieve stride rates of up to 4.6 strides per second, while women reach 4.8 strides per second. The distance required for acceleration varies between sex and maximum-speed ability. In general, men tend to reach maximum speed at 60 to 80 meters; for women, this typically occurs at 50 to 60 meters. Additionally, athletes with a high maximum speed require a longer distance to achieve their top speed, therefore achieving it later in the sprint, resulting in a longer acceleration stage compared to slower athletes. While the acceleration phase is relatively long, it must be remembered that at each distance, a high speed relative to the maximum speed is achieved. Usain Bolt, for example, during his Olympic gold medal performance in Beijing achieved 73 percent of his maximal velocity at 10 meters, 85 percent at 20 meters, 93 percent at 30 meters, and 96 percent at 40 meters.

Eventually, an athlete reaches the maximum-speed phase, or the point at which acceleration is no longer possible. At this point, the athlete has achieved maximal velocity, which is typically 11 or more meters per second for elite women sprinters and 12 or more meters per second for elite male sprinters. Further acceleration at this point is limited by short ground contact times and, hence, the inability to exert additional forces. Here an athlete typically covers 20 to 30 meters. Once athletes reach this point, they should no longer try to accelerate and instead focus on maintaining maximum speed.

The final stage is where an athlete is unable to hold maximal speed and enters a phase of deceleration. Despite the fact that some athletes appear to speed up at this phase, the reality is that they are simply maintaining their speed to a greater extent than other athletes. The length of this phase depends on the acceleration pattern, the athlete's conditioning level, and loss of technique caused by race pressure. Athletes who have a longer acceleration phase to top speed have an advantage in this phase because they have been required to hold maximum speed for a shorter distance. A feature of modern sprinting is that athletes are showing an increased ability to hold high speeds during this phase so that deceleration today plays a smaller role in the final phase of a 100-meter sprint.

The figures stated earlier represent the patterns for elite sprinters, and this analysis is inappropriate for classifying the sprint components for youth athletes, recreational athletes, and even sub-elite athletes who are likely to reach their maximum speed earlier and, thus, have a far greater degree of deceleration. Very young athletes, for example, may achieve top speed at 20 meters, maintain this for perhaps 5 meters, and then decelerate for the remaining 75 meters of the race.

In considering the 200- and 400-meter sprints, the acceleration stage of those races is purposely lengthened. Unlike the 100 meters, where in most cases the athletes aim to accelerate maximally to achieve top speed as soon as possible,

200-meter and 400-meter sprinters control their acceleration (partly because of race strategy and because of starting on the curve of the track) and extend the absolute length of this acceleration component. It is always a challenge for a sprinter to try to run at top speed in a curve. Therefore, the acceleration to maximum speed in the longer sprints is influenced by the lane the athlete is running in (the inner few lanes providing the greatest challenge), his or her ability to run the curve, and the particular race strategy. This results in a large range of race profiles for the acceleration, maximum speed, and speed endurance components and their distribution for athletes in the 200 and 400 meters.

TRACK-SPECIFIC DRILLS

Given the vital role of speed in track sprinting, the majority of the technical models (chapter 2) for sprinting emanate from track and field. Similarly, the majority of the techniques outlined in chapter 3 have their basis in track sprinting. Therefore, the drills presented in chapter 3 play a vital role in the development of appropriate technique for a track sprinter. Coaches and athletes can select drills that relate specifically to the technical aspects of acceleration and maximum-speed running along with exercises associated with the application of acceleration and maximum-speed abilities. Rather than repeat these exercises, this section examines two elements that are unique to track: starting from blocks and sprinting the curve.

Starting From the Blocks

In track sprinting, block clearance is the first component of the acceleration phase. In response to the starter's pistol, athletes must clear the blocks to begin their acceleration. Block starts should be included and taught to athletes who have developed fundamental competency in basic acceleration technique. In the initial stages of development, starts from lying, standing, and three points can develop the fundamentals of starting so that the more complex skill of starting from blocks can be introduced on a sound foundation. (See the sprint from ground, sprint from three-point stance, and fall-in sprint drills in chapter 3.)

The specific block position that athletes use varies somewhat based on their technical style and competency, body size, preferences, and strength. However, in general, when in the set position, an athlete's front knee angle should at least be 90 degrees, and rear knee angle should be at least 120 degrees (see figure 6.1). The spacing of the hands is particularly important. Many young athletes adopt a very wide spacing, mimicking the style of physically mature top sprinters, but they often lack the strength required to clear the blocks effectively from this position and should use a narrower width between the hands to better support the torso and to maintain a higher center of gravity.

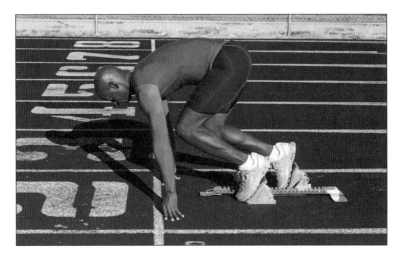

Figure 6.1 Proper set position for starting from blocks.

Improper hand spacing is easily identified by errors such as ineffective initial movement through the upper body when trying to clear the blocks, breaking at the elbows, dipping the upper torso, and immediately standing up once clearing the blocks. What the coach should see is an efficient and explosive movement from the hands as the legs drive rearward against the blocks, resulting in the straight-line posture outlined in chapter 2.

Stronger athletes can adopt a more acute torso angle to allow for greater explosive extension through the hip and torso. Using a wide hand placement, leaning forward over the start line, and dropping the head, which lowers the shoulders relative to the hips, can all create a more acute torso angle in stronger, more powerful athletes (see figure 6.2).

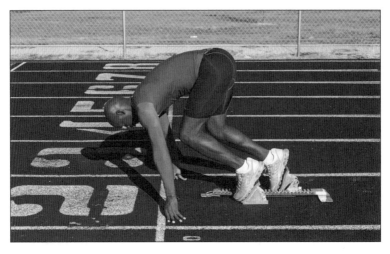

Figure 6.2 Set position with a more acute torso angle.

Starting and Running on the Curve

A critical aspect of sprinting in the 200- and 400-meter races is the ability to start and accelerate and sprint effectively on the curve. Again, similar to introducing block starts, the coach should not emphasize this too early in the development of a young sprinter at the expense of fundamental technique. For example, incorporating block starts on the bend (as in the 200 and 400 meters) with an athlete who has yet to develop basic technique in acceleration and block technique may inhibit the longer-term development of the athlete's sprinting.

Accelerating and sprinting on a curve is primarily characterized by a body lean and, of course, increased forces to both overcome gravity and also to provide centripetal acceleration to negotiate the curve without drifting to the outside if the lane. Athletes should try to run on the inside of the lane around the curve as this is the shortest distance. The degree to which athletes are angled to the track depends on the lane they run in and the speed at which they run. In terms of the lane used, inside lanes require a sharper turn than outside lanes but involve less total distance in the curve. Inside lanes therefore require greater angles of lean to overcome these sharper turns and greater centripetal forces. In terms of the speed at which the athlete is running, the greater the speed, the greater the body lean required to overcome the increased inertial forces, where the body's ideal motion would be to continue in a straight line.

The body lean that the athlete employs should initiate from the ground and not merely be the athlete tilting to the left at the waist (see figure 6.3). A lean from the ground allows effective force production while running the curve. As

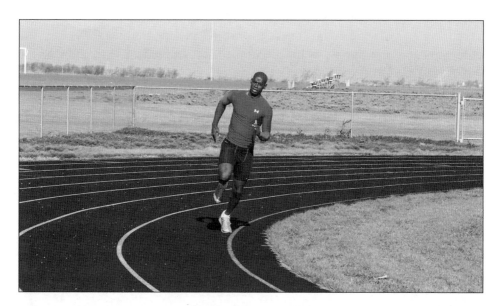

Figure 6.3   Inward lean from the ground.

athletes negotiate the curve, the left stride is shorter than the right, and athletes use a shorter stride length in general when running a curve (but spend more time on the ground to apply force). The right arm swing often crosses toward or beyond the midline to assist with centripetal acceleration and lift.

Sprinting on the curve is less mechanically efficient than sprinting in a straight line. Athletes cannot sprint as fast on a curve as they can on the straight because of the necessity to counteract inertial forces. The ideal technique minimizes potential loss of force in negotiating the curve and optimizes acceleration and speed through the techniques mentioned. Sprinters should exit the curve in a position that allows them to continue increasing their speed as they reach the straight portion of the track. For this reason, sprinters must control their body position. A common error in this regard is allowing the left shoulder to open to the inside of the track instead of maintaining a strong posture to apply force. Another error is to overstride in the curve.

SPRINT TRAINING PROGRAM BASICS

Considering the magnitude of the effect a sprint training session has on the body and the other development factors involved in sprint training, sequencing the training for sprinters is important. Although long-term periodization for sprinters is not within the scope of this chapter, it is helpful to outline general trends and principles in planning sessions.

Table 6.4 outlines sprint training sessions within a training week for a developing (e.g., high school) sprinter. Table 6.5 outlines these sessions for a collegiate sprinter. For the developing sprinter, a greater emphasis is placed on building the fundamental skills required of track and field and general athletic development, and the program uses the practices outlined in chapter 3 to ensure development of appropriate technical competency. The collegiate sprinter, on the other hand, performs sessions with a greater specificity of focus. In other words, the developing sprinter is still *learning how to sprint* and gain conditioning. The elite sprinter in this example is focusing on specific aspects of *race execution*.

Table 6.4 Sample Training Week for a Middle School or High School Sprinter

Day	Session type	Activities*	Strength and conditioning
Monday	Track session	Bounds: (4-6 × 40 m) Acceleration from 3-point start: (5-6 × 20 m)	None
Tuesday	Tempo session	On-grass runs: 6-7 × 100 m at 70% effort A series of runs focusing on relaxing at speed The grass surface reduces the impact stress on the body	Introduction to general strength and conditioning
Wednesday	Cross-training	Other sports or off	None
Thursday	Track session	Basic drills: standing arm swing, ankling, marching A, wall drive (single exchange), step over Acceleration-speed from standing: 4-5 × 40 m	Introduction to general strength and conditioning
Friday	Cross-training	Other sports or off	None
Saturday	Track session	Speed endurance: 3 × 200 m at 85% of maximal speed and 3 min. between repetitions	Introduction to general strength and conditioning
Sunday	Off	Off	Off

*Activities outlined are in addition to a warm-up and preparatory activities. Tempo running is generally done at 65-75% of maximum velocity, with an emphasis on maintaining smooth running form. All distances include a walk-back of equal distances.

Table 6.5 Sample Training Week for a Collegiate Sprinter

Day	Session type	Activities*	Strength and conditioning	Other activity
Monday	Track session	Run-throughs: 5 × 80 m Blocks/ accelerations: 5 × 20 m and 4 × 30 m	Ballistic and maximal strength: lower body Olympic lifting	
Tuesday	Tempo session	On-grass runs: 6 × 100 m, 4 × 150 m	None	
Wednesday	Plyometrics	80-120 foot contacts Depth jumps Hops Medicine ball drills Speed bounding	None	Aquatic: recovery session
Thursday	Track session	Run-throughs: 5 × 60 m Speed, from standing: 4 × 30 m, 1 × 50 m	Ballistic and maximal strength: upper body	
Friday	Tempo session	On grass runs: 2 × 100 m, 2 × 150 m, 1 × 200 m	Ballistic and maximal strength: lower body Olympic lifting (to be performed before the tempo session)	
Saturday	Track session	Speed-Endurance: 2-3 × 150 m with 3-min. recovery between repetitions	None	Massage
Sunday	Off	Off	Off	Off

*Activities outlined are in addition to a warm-up and preparatory activities. Tempo running is generally done at 65-75% of maximum velocity, with an emphasis on maintaining smooth running form. All distances include a walk-back of equal distances.

References

Chapter 1

Deacon, J. 2011. Acceleration: theory and practice. *Professional Strength and Conditioning Journal* 21: 16–21.

Goodwin, J. 2011. Maximum velocity is when we can no longer accelerate. *Professional Strength and Conditioning Journal* 21: 3–9.

Jeffreys, I. 2006a. A motor development approach to enhancing agility. Part 1. *Strength and Conditioning Journal* 28 (5): 72–76.

Jeffreys, I. 2006b. A motor development approach to enhancing agility. Part 2. *Strength and Conditioning Journal* 28 (6): 10–14.

Jeffreys, I. 2006c. Optimising speed and agility development using target classifications and motor control principles. Part 1. *Professional Strength and Conditioning Journal* 3: 11–14.

Jeffreys, I. 2006d. Optimising speed and agility development using target classifications and motor control principles. Part 2. *Professional Strength and Conditioning Journal* 4: 12–17.

Jeffreys, I. 2007. *Total soccer fitness.* Monterrey, CA: Coaches Choice.

Jeffreys, I. 2009. *Gamespeed: movement training for superior sports performance.* Monterrey, CA: Coaches Choice.

McGinnis, P.M. 2005. *Biomechanics of sport and exercise.* 2d ed. Champaign, IL: Human Kinetics.

Weyand, P.G., D.B. Sternlight, M.J. Bellizzi, and S. Wright S. 2000. Faster top running speeds are achieved with greater ground forces not more rapid leg movements. *Journal of Applied Physiology* 89 (5): 1991–1999.

Weyand, P.G., and J.A. Davis. 2005. Running performance has a structural basis. *The Journal of Experimental Biology* 208: 2625–2631.

Weyand, P.G., R.F. Sandell, D.N. Prime, and M.W. Bundle. 2010. The biological limits to running speed are imposed from the ground up. *Journal of Applied Physiology* (Apr) 108 (4): 950–961.

Chapter 2

Baker, D. 1999. A comparison of running speed and quickness between elite professional and young rugby league players. *Strength and Conditioning Coach* 7 (3): 3–7.

Docherty, D., H.A. Wenger, and P. Neary. 1998. Time–motion analysis related to the physiological demands of rugby. *Journal of Human Movement Studies* 14: 269–277.

Gambetta V. 1996. How to develop sport–specific speed. *Sports Coach* 19 (3): 22–24.

Gambetta V. 2007. *Athletic development.* Champaign, IL: Human Kinetics.

Sayers M. 2000. Running techniques for field sport players. *Sports Coach* Autumn: 26–27.

Sheppard, J.M., and W. Young. 2006. Agility literature review: classifications, training and testing. *Journal of Sport Sciences* 24 (9): 919–932.

Chapter 3

Baechle, T.R. 1994. *Essentials of strength training and conditioning.* Champaign, IL: Human Kinetics.

Baker, D. and S. Nance. 1999. The relationship between running speed and measures of strength and power in professional rugby league players. *Journal of Strength and Conditioning Research* 13 (3): 230–235.

Balyi, I. 1995. Long term athlete development. *Strength and Conditioning Coach* 3 (2): 10–14.

Balyi, I. 1996. *Planing for training and performance.* Vancouver, Canada: BC Sports Services Branch.

Blazevich, T. 1997a. Resistance training for sprinters. Part 1. *Strength and Conditioning Coach* 4 (3): 9–12.

Blazevich, T. 1997b. Resistance training for sprinters. Part 2. *Strength and Conditioning Coach* 5 (1): 5–10.

Bobbert, M.F. 1990. Drop jumping as a training method for jumping ability. *Sports Medicine* 9 (1): 7–22.

Brown, L.E. and V.A. Ferrigno. 2005. *Training for speed, agility, and quickness.* Champaign, IL: Human Kinetics.

Brughelli, M., J. Cronin, and K. Nosaka. Forthcoming. Muscle architecture and optimum angle of the knee flexors and extensors: a comparison between cyclists and Australian rules football players. *Journal of Strength and Conditioning Research.*

Clutch, D. and M. Wilton. 1983. The effect of depth jumps and weight training on leg strength and vertical jump. 54:5–10.

Dintiman, G. and B. Ward. 2003. *Sports speed.* 3d ed. Champaign, IL: Human Kinetics.

Donati, A. 1996. The association between the development of strength and speed. *New Studies in Athletics* 2 (3): 51–58.

Faccioni, A. Modern Speed Training. In: Faccioni; Oztrack E–books. 2003. p. E–book.

Francis, C. 1997. *Training for speed.* Canberra, Australian Capital Territory: Faccioni Speed & Conditioning Consultants.

Francis, C. 2005. Speed training. Francis speed training seminar, Vancouver, Canada.

Gambetta, V. 1990. Speed development for football. *National Strength and Conditioning Association Journal* 12 (1): 45–46.

Gambetta, V. 1996. How to develop sport–specific speed. *Sports Coach* 19 (3): 22–24.

Gambetta, V. 2007. *Athletic development: the art and science of functional sports conditioning.* Champaign, IL: Human Kinetics.

Hakkinen, K. and P.V. Komi. 1985. Effect of explosive type strength training on electromyographic and force production characteristics of leg extensor muscles during concentric and various stretch–shortening cycle exercises. *Scandanavian Journal of Sports Sciences* 7 (2): 65–76.

Harrison, A.J. and B. Gillian. 2009. The effect of resisted sprint training on speed and strength performance in male rugby players. *Journal of Strength and Conditioning Research* 23 (1): 275–283.

Knicker, A.J. 1994. Untersuchungen zur ubereinstimmung von zugwiderstandslaufen und sprintbewegungen. Paper presented at the Widerstandbelastungen im Schnelligkeitstraining, Koln, Germany.

Knicker, A.J. 1997. Neuromechanics of sprint–specific training skills. Paper presented at the 15 International Symposium on Biomechanics in Sport, Denton, Texas.

Kunz, H. and D.A. Kaufmann, 1981. Biomechanics of hill sprinting. *Track Technique* 82: 2603–2605.

Kyrolainen, H., P. Komi, and A. Belli. 1999. Changes in muscle activity patterns and kinetics with increasing running speed. *Journal of Strength and Conditioning Research* 13 (4): 400–406.

Letzelter, M., G. Sauerwein, and R. Burger. 1994. Resistance runs in speed development. *Modern Athlete and Coach* 22: 20–29.

Lidor, R. and Y. Meckel. 2004. Physiological, skill development and motor learning considerations for 100 metres. *New Studies in Athletics* 19 (1): 7–12.

Luchtenbern, B. 1990. Training for running. *Science Periodical of Research and Technology in Sport* 10 (3): 1–6.

Mann, R.V. 1981. A kinetic analysis of sprinting. *Medicine and Science in Sports and Exercise* 13 (5): 325–328.

Maulder, P.S., E.J. Bradshaw, and J. Keogh. 2008. Kinematic alterations due to different loading schemes in early acceleration sprint performance from starting blocks. *Journal of Strength and Conditioning Research* 22 (6): 1992–2002.

Mero, A. and P. Komi. 1985. Effects of supramaximal velocity on biomechanical variables in sprinting. *International Journal of Sport Biomechanics* 1: 240–252.

Mouchbahani, R., A. Gollhofer, and H. Dickhuth. 2004. Pulley systems in sprint training. *Modern Athlete and Coach* 42 (3): 14–17.

National Strength and Conditioning Association. Dawes. J. and M. Roozen, eds. 2012a *Developing agility and quickness.* Champaign, IL: Human Kinetics.

National Strength and Conditioning Association. Reuter, B., ed. 2012b. *Developing endurance.* Champaign, IL: Human Kinetics.

Saraslandis, P. 2000. Maximum speed: flat running or resistance training. *New Studies in Athletics* 3 (4): 45–51.

Sheppard, J. 2003. Strength and conditioning exercise selection in speed development. *Strength and Conditioning Journal* 25 (4): 26–30.

Sheppard, J. 2004. The use of resisted and assisted training methods for speed development: coaching considerations. *Modern Athlete and Coach* 42 (4): 9–13.

Sheppard, J. and G. Sleivert. 2005. Use of resistance with sprint training. *Sports Coach* 28 (3): 14–15.

Sheppard, J.M., D. Chapman, C. Gough, M. McGuigan, and R.U. Newton. 2008a. The association between changes in vertical jump and changes in strength and power qualities in elite volleyball players over 1 year. Paper presented at the National Strength and Conditioning Association Annual Conference. Abstract in the *Journal of Strength and Conditioning Research* 22 (6): 1–115.

Sheppard, J.M., M.R. McGuigan, and R.U. Newton. 2008b. The effects of depth–jumping on vertical jump performance of elite volleyball players: an examination of the transfer of increased stretch–load tolerance to spike jump performance. *Journal of Australian Strength and Conditioning* 16 (4): 3–10.

Spinks, C.D., A.J. Murphy, W. L. Spinks, and R.G. Lockie. 2007. The effects of resisted sprint training on acceleration performance and kinematics in soccer, rugby union, and Australian football players. *Journal of Strength and Conditioning Research* 21 (1): 77–85.

Tziortzis, S. and G.P. Paradisis. 1996. The effect of sprint resisted training on the peak anaerobic power and 60 m performance. Paper presented at the Frontiers in Sport Science May 28–31, Nice, France.

Vonstein, W. 1994. Kritische betrachtung des zugwiderstainings. Paper presented at the Widerstandsbelastungen im Schnelligkeitstaining, Koln, Germany.

Young, W.B., B. McLean, and J. Ardagna. 1995. Relationship between strength qualities and sprinting performance. *Journal of Sports Medicine and Physical Fitness* 35 (1): 13–19.

Zatsiorsky, V.M. and W.J. Kraemer. 2006. *Science and practice of strength training.* 2d ed. Champaign, IL: Human Kinetics.

Chapter 4

Altug, Z., T. Altug, and A. Altug. 1987. A test selection guide for assessing and evaluating athletes. *NSCA Journal* 9 (3): 67–69.

American Alliance for Health, Physical Education, Recreation and Dance. 1980. *AAHPERD Health-related fitness test*. Reston, VA: Author.

Anderson, J.C. 2005. Stretching before and after exercise. Effect on muscle soreness and injury risk. *Journal of Athletic Training* 40 (3): 218–220.

Arthur, M., and B. Bailey. 1998. *Complete conditioning for football*. Champaign, IL: Human Kinetics.

Barnes, M., and J.M. Cissik. 2008. *Training for the 40-yard dash*. Monterey, CA: Coaches Choice.

Baumgartner, T., and A. Jackson. 1987. *Measurement for evaluation in physical education and exercise science*. Dubuque, IA: Brown.

Bridgman, R. 1991. A coaches' guide to testing for athletic attributes. *NSCA Journal*. 13 (3): 34–36.

Cissik, J.M., and M. Barnes. 2004. *Sport speed and agility*. Monterey, CA: Coaches Choice.

Fleck, S. 1983. Interval: physiological basis. *NSCA Journal* 5 (5): 40.

Flexibility: Roundtable. 1984. *NSCA Journal* 6 (4): 10–22, 71–73.

Funk, D.C., A.M. Swank, B.M. Mikala, T.A. Fagan, and B.K. Farr. 2003. Impact of prior exercise on hamstring flexibility: a comparison of proprioceptive neuromuscular facilitation and static stretching. *The Journal of Strength and Conditioning Research* 17 (3): 489–492.

Graham, J. 1994. Guidelines for providing valid testing of athletes' fitness levels. *Strength and Conditioning Journal* 16 (6): 7–14.

Graham, J., and V. Ferrigno. 2005. Agility and balance training. In *Training for speed, agility, and quickness*. 2d ed. Ed. L.E. Brown and V.A. Ferrigno. Champaign, IL: Human Kinetics.

Harman, E. 2008. Principles of test selection and administration. In *Essentials of strength training and conditioning*. 3d ed. Ed. T.R. Baechle, R.W. Earle, and National Strength and Conditioning Association. Champaign, IL: Human Kinetics.

Hastad, D.N., and A.C. Lacy. 1989. *Measurement and evaluation in contemporary physical education*. Scottsdale, AZ: Gousch.

Hoffman, J.R. 2002. *Physiological aspects of sport training and performance*. Champaign, IL: Human Kinetics.

Hoffman, J.R. 2006. *Norms for fitness, performance, and health*. Champaign, IL: Human Kinetics.

Hoffman, J.R., S. Epstein, M. Einbinder, and Y. Weinstein. 1999. The influence of aerobic capacity on anaerobic performance and recovery indices in basketball players. *The Journal of Strength and Conditioning Research* 13: 407–411.

Hopkins, C. 1980. *Understanding educational research*. Columbus, OH: Merrill.

Howley, E.T., and B.D. Franks. 2003. *Health fitness instructor's handbook*, 4th ed. Champaign, IL: Human Kinetics.

Jeffreys, I. 2008. Warm-up and stretching. In *Essentials of strength training and conditioning*. 3d ed. Ed. T.R. Baechle, R.W. Earle, and National Strength and Conditioning Association. Champaign, IL: Human Kinetics.

Johnson, B., and J. Nelson. 1986. Practical measurement for evaluation in physical education. 4th ed., New York: Macmillan.

Kirkendall, D.T. 2000. Physiology of soccer. In *Exercise and sport science*. Ed. W.E. Garrett and D.T. Kirkendall. Philadelphia, PA: Lippincott, Williams and Wilkins.

Kontor, K. 1981. Testing and evaluation. *NSCA Journal* 3 (2): 7.

Kraemer, W.J., and L.A. Gotshalk. 2000. Physiology of American football. In *Exercise and sport science*. Ed. W.E. Garrett and D.T. Kirkendall. Philadelphia, PA: Lippincott, Williams and Wilkins.

Lentz, D., and A. Hardyk. 2005. Speed training. In *Training for speed, agility, and quickness*. 2d ed. Ed. L.E. Brown and V.A. Ferrigno. Champaign, IL: Human Kinetics.

Lund, H., P. Vestergaard–Poulsen, I.L. Kanstrup, and P. Sejrsen. 1998. The effect of passive stretching on delayed onset muscle soreness, and other detrimental effects following eccentric exercise. *Scandinavian Journal of Medicine and Science in Sports* 8 (4): 216–221.

Prentice, W.E. 1983. A comparison of static stretching and PNF stretching for improving hip joint flexibility. *Athletic Training* 18 (1): 56–59.

Semenick, D. 1984. Anaerobic testing: practical applications. *NSCA Journal* 6 (5): 45.

Vestegen, M. 2004. *Core performance*. Emmaus, PA: Rodale Press.

Chapter 5

Jeffreys, I. 2006a. A motor development approach to enhancing agility. Part 1. *Strength and Conditioning Journal* 28 (5): 72–76.

Jeffreys, I. 2006b. A motor development approach to enhancing agility. Part 2. *Strength and Conditioning Journal* 28 (6): 10–14.

Jeffreys, I. 2006c. Optimising speed and agility development using target classifications and motor control principles. Part 1. *Professional Strength and Conditioning Journal*.

Jeffreys, I. 2006d. Optimising speed and agility development using target classifications and motor control principles. Part 2. *Professional Strength and Conditioning Journal*.

Jeffreys, I. 2007. *Total soccer fitness*. Monterrey, CA: Coaches Choice.

Jeffreys, I. 2009. *Gamespeed: movement training for superior sports performance*. Monterrey, CA: Coaches Choice.

Chapter 6

Baseball

Coleman, A.E. 2000. *52–week baseball training*. Champaign, IL: Human Kinetics.

Coleman, A.E. 2009. In–season base running speed drills. Unpublished manuscript.

Coleman, A.E., and Dupler, T.L. 2004. Changes in running speed in game situations during a season of major league baseball. *Journal of Exercise Physiology online* 7 (3): 89–93.

Coleman, A.E., and Dupler, T.L. 2005. Differences in running speed among major league players in game situations. *Journal of Exercise Physiology online* 8 (2): 10–15.

Coleman, A.E., and Lasky, L. 1992. Assessing running speed and body composition in professional baseball players. *Journal of Applied Sport Science Research* 6: 2007–2213.

Cronin, R. 2009. Game speed training in baseball. *Journal of Strength and Conditioning Research* 31 (2): 13–25.

Gambetta, V. 2007. *Athletic development: The art and science of functional sports conditioning*. Champaign, IL: Human Kinetics.

Spaniol, F.J. 2005. Body composition and baseball performance. *NSCA Performance Training Journal* 4(1): 10–11.

Spaniol, F.J. 2007. Physiological characteristics of NAIA intercollegiate baseball players [abstract]. *Journal of Strength and Conditioning Research* 21 (4): e25.

Spaniol, F.J., D. Melrose, M. Bohling, and R, Bonnette. 2005. Physiological characteristics of NCAA Division I baseball players [abstract]. *Journal of Strength and Conditioning Research* 19 (4): e34.

Ice Hockey

Lentz, D., and A. Hardyk. 2005. Speed training. In *Training for speed, agility, and quickness*. 2d ed. Ed. Brown, L.E. and V.A. Ferrigno. Champaign, IL: Human Kinetics.

Manners, T.W. 2004. Sport–specific training for ice hockey. *Strength and Conditioning Journal* 26(2): 16–22.

Warren, Y.B., M.H. McDowell, and B.J. Scarlett. 2001. Specificity of sprint and agility training methods. *The Journal of Strength and Conditioning Research* 15(3): 315–319.

Rugby

Jeffreys, I. 2006a. A motor development approach to enhancing agility. Part 1. *Strength and Conditioning Journal* 28 (5): 72–76.

Jeffreys, I. 2006b. A motor development approach to enhancing agility. Part 2. *Strength and Conditioning Journal* 28 (6): 10–14.

Jeffreys, I. 2006c. Optimising speed and agility development using target classifications and motor control principles. Part 1. *Professional Strength and Conditioning Journal* 3: 11–14.

Jeffreys, I. 2006d. Optimising speed and agility development using target classifications and motor control principles. Part 2. *Professional Strength and Conditioning Journal* 4: 12–17.

Jeffreys, I. 2007. Warm–up revisited: The ramp method of optimizing warm–ups. *Professional Strength and Conditioning Journal* 6: 12–18.

Jeffreys, I. 2009. *Gamespeed: movement training for superior sports performance*. Monterey, CA: Coaches Choice.

Soccer

Jeffreys, I. 2006a. A motor development approach to enhancing agility. Part 1. *Strength and Conditioning Journal* 28 (5): 72–76.

Jeffreys, I. 2006b. A motor development approach to enhancing agility. Part 2. *Strength and Conditioning Journal* 28 (6): 10–14.

Jeffreys, I. 2006c. Optimising speed and agility development using target classifications and motor control principles. Part 1. *Professional Strength and Conditioning* 3: 11–14.

Jeffreys, I. 2006d. Optimising speed and agility development using target classifications and motor control principles. Part 2. *Professional Strength and Conditioning* 4: 12–17.

Jeffreys, I. 2007a. *Total soccer fitness*. Monterey, CA: Coaches Choice.

Jeffreys, I. 2007b. Warm–up revisited: The RAMP method of optimizing warm–ups. *Professional Strength and Conditioning* 6: 12–18.

Jeffreys, I. 2008. Movement training for field sports: soccer. *Strength and Conditioning Journal*. 30 (4): 19–27.

Jeffreys, I. 2009. *Gamespeed: movement training for superior sports performance*. Monterey, CA: Coaches Choice.

Tennis

Baechle, T., and Earle, R. 2008. *Essentials of strength training and conditioning*. 3d ed. Champaign, IL: Human Kinetics.

Brown, L. ed. 2005. *Speed, agility, and quickness*. Champaign, IL: Human Kinetics.

Crotin, R. 2009. Game speed training in baseball. *Strength and Conditioning Journal* 31: 13–25.

Dawes, J. 2008. Creating open agility drills. *Strength and Conditioning Journal* 30: 54–55.

Flannagan, E., and P. Comyns. 2008. The use of contact time and the reactive strength index to optimize fast stretch–shortening cycle training. *Strength and Conditioning Journal* 30: 32–38.

Hansen, K., and J. Cronin. 2009. Training loads for the development of the lower body. *Strength and Conditioning Journal* 31: 17–33.

Kovacs, M. 2004. Energy system–specific training for tennis. *Strength and Conditioning Journal* 26: 10–13.

Kovacs, M. 2009. Movement for tennis: the importance of lateral training. *Strength and Conditioning Journal* 30: 77–85.

Kovacs, M. et al. 2008. Efficient deceleration: the forgotten factor in tennis–specific training. *Strength and Conditioning Journal* 30: 58–69.

Matsuda T. et al. 2005. Quick movement in footwork: effectiveness of the split–step. *Proceedings of the Annual Meeting of Japanese Society for Othopaedic Biomechanics* 26: 363–367.

Ochi, S., and M.J. Campbell. 2009. The progressive physical development of a high–performance tennis player. *Strength and Conditioning Journal* 31: 59–68.

Pankhurst, A. 2006. The progressive development of a high–performance tennis player. *USTA High Performance Coaching* 8: 1–9.

Roetert, E.P., and T.S. Ellenbecker. 2001. Biomechanics of tennis movements. *International Tennis Federation CSSR* 24: 15–17.

Roetert, E.P., M. Kovacs, D. Knudson, and J.L. Groppel. 2005. Biomechanics of the tennis ground-strokes. *Strength and Conditioning Journal* 31 (4): 41–49.

Zatsiorsky, V., and W. Kramer. 2007. *Science and practice of strength training.* Champaign, IL: Human Kinetics.

Index

Note: The italicized *f* and *t* following page numbers refer to figures and tables, respectively.

About the NSCA

The **National Strength and Conditioning Association (NSCA)** is the world's leading organization in the field of sport conditioning. Drawing on the resources and expertise of the most recognized professionals in strength training and conditioning, sport science, performance research, education, and sports medicine, the NSCA is the world's trusted source of knowledge and training guidelines for coaches and athletes. The NSCA provides the crucial link between the lab and the field.

About the Editor

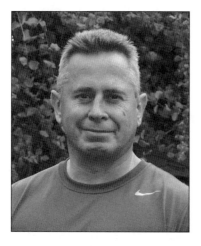

Ian Jeffreys has established himself as one of the most respected strength and conditioning coaches in the UK. He has been the strength and conditioning coach for the Welsh Schools national rugby team and has worked with athletes, clubs, and sport organizations, from junior level to professional level, around the world.

Ian is currently a reader in strength and conditioning at the University of South Wales, and also is the Proprietor of All-Pro Performance, a performance enhancement company based in Brecon Wales. He has been a member of the National Strength and Conditioning Association (NSCA) since 1989. He is a certified strength and conditioning specialist (CSCS) and certified personal trainer (NSCA-CPT) with the NSCA, and he has been recertified with distinction (*D) in both categories. He is also a registered strength and conditioning coach—recertified with distinction. Ian currently sits on the NSCA High School Executive Committee and was the NSCA's High School Professional of the Year in 2006, the first time the award was presented to a coach working outside the United States, and was made a fellow of the NSCA in 2009.

Ian is on the British Olympic Association register of strength and conditioning professionals. He is a director of the United Kingdom Strength and Conditioning Association, where he is an accredited strength and conditioning coach (ASCC) and an assessor for the organization. He is also a lead tutor for the UKSCA education workshops.

Ian has authored numerous strength and conditioning articles that have been featured in leading international journals. He is the editor of the UKSCA journal *Professional Strength and Conditioning* and is on the editorial board for the NSCA's *Strength and Conditioning Journal* and the *Journal of Australian Strength and Conditioning.* Ian has authored three books and the warm-up and stretching chapter for the third edition of *Essentials of Strength Training and Conditioning.*

Ian is a sought-after presenter and has given keynote presentations and hosted high-performance workshops at major conferences around the world. His specialty is speed and agility development.

About the Contributors

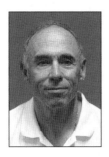

Al Biancani, EdD, CSCS*D, is the head strength and conditioning coach for the Chinese women's national basketball team and holds the same position for the under 17 and 18 boys and girls national basketball teams. Before his current position, Biancani was the head strength and conditioning coach of the NBA's Sacramento Kings for 18 seasons and also the WNBA's Sacramento Monarchs, who won the 2005 championship. Biancani has spent more than four decades in the strength and conditioning field, having earned a BS and an MS in physical education from California State University, and he also earned an EdD in physical education and sociology from Utah State University. Biancani is a certified strength and conditioning coach with distinction from the National Strength and Conditioning Association and has contributed to numerous strength and conditioning books and publications both internationally and in the United States. He has presented workshops, clinics, and camps all over the world. Biancani and his wife, Shirong Tao, have three children and four grandchildren.

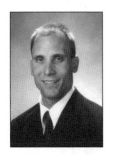

John Graham, MS, HFS, CSCS*D, RSCC*D, FNSCA, is the director of Sports and Human Performance at St. Luke's University Health Network in Allentown and Bethlehem, Pa. Graham is an adjunct professor at the College of New Jersey in the Department of Health and Exercise Science and is a member of the Industry Advisory Panel for the American Council on Exercise. He serves as an associate editor for the National Strength and Conditioning Association's *Strength and Conditioning Journal*. Graham is the current chair of the National Strength and Conditioning Association (NSCA) certification committee. He is an NSCA fellow, certified strength and conditioning specialist, registered strength and conditioning coach, and American College of Sports Medicine certified health and fitness specialist. He served as a member of the NSCA Board of Directors from 2001 to 2003 and served as vice president in 2002 and secretary/treasurer in 2003. Graham was awarded the NSCA *Strength and Conditioning Journal* Editorial Excellence Award in 2000. He has authored or contributed to local, regional, and national peer-reviewed and lay publications on health, fitness, and sport conditioning and has given local, regional, national, and international presentations on health, fitness, and sport conditioning. Graham is married to Lisa and has two daughters, Lindsey and Alexas.

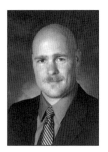

Jeff Kipp, MS, CSCS, serves as an assistant strength and conditioning coach at the U.S. Air Force Academy, supervising the speed, strength, and conditioning program for the hockey team. He has also supervised speed development for the Falcon football team, served as the primary strength and conditioning coach for the lacrosse program, and worked with the track and field and cross country teams. Kipp served as a performance coach at Velocity Sports Performance in Denver and Evergreen, Colo. He also served as an assistant strength and conditioning coach at the University of Denver and the strength and conditioning coordinator at the Colorado School of Mines. Kipp holds strength and conditioning specialist credentials through the National Strength and Conditioning Association (NSCA) and is certified through the National Association of Speed and Explosion, where he serves as the director for Colorado. He is a member of the Collegiate Strength and Conditioning Coaches Association, USA Weightlifting, and USA Track and Field. As a speaker for the NSCA, Kipp addresses groups of national and international coaches on strength training, speed development, and conditioning. He has authored several text chapters and served on the review board for text chapters by other strength and conditioning authors.

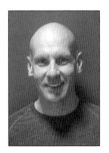

Jeremy Sheppard, PhD, CSCS, serves as the sport science manager and head of strength and conditioning at the Hurley Surfing Australia High Performance Centre. He is also a senior lecturer for Edith Cowan University.

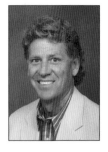

Frank Spaniol, EdD, CSCS*D, FNSCA, serves as professor of kinesiology at Texas A&M University at Corpus Christi, where he teaches sport science and directs the Sport Science Research Laboratory. Spaniol has published and presented extensively in applied sport science and recently coauthored an e-text, *Dynamic Biomechanics*. In addition, he has served as an NCAA Division I head baseball coach, worked with numerous Major League Baseball organizations, and has been awarded a fellowship by the National Strength and Conditioning Association (NSCA).

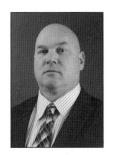

Mark D. Stephenson, MS, ATC, CSCS*D, has more than 23 years of experience working in the human performance field. He serves as the director of the Human Performance Program at a special operations unit for the Department of Defense (DoD). Before working with the DoD, Mark was the director of the Human Performance Center at the National Strength and Conditioning Association (NSCA), where he developed the Tactical Strength and Conditioning program. While at the NSCA, he also served as the head strength and conditioning coach for Colorado College's men's ice hockey team and the tactical physiologist for the Colorado Springs Police Department's SWAT team. Mark came to the NSCA by way of Providence College, where he served as head strength and conditioning coach. Stephenson started his career in human performance as an athletic trainer, working in a sports medicine clinic with orthopedic surgeons and serving as the head athletic trainer at a high school. Throughout his career in human performance he has worked at various athletic levels, including high school, collegiate Division I, Olympic, and professional.

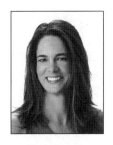

Diane Vives is owner and director of Vives Training Systems and Fit4Austin in Austin, Texas. She is a strength and conditioning specialist who serves a wide range of athletes and clients in the Austin community. She is an internationally recognized presenter who provides integration strategies for current and evidence-based fitness and training techniques and tools. She is passionate about targeting the needs of the female athlete and creating resources for creating the best comprehensive approach to elevate female athletic performance and reduce injury risk in sports and fitness. She serves on the Under Armour Performance Training Council. She is a regular contributing author and expert for several national and regional publications and is a contributing member of the Functional Movement Systems team. With 15 years of experience, she is a strength training specialist and professional mentor, who shares her knowledge, experience, and resources on her website www.dianevives.com.

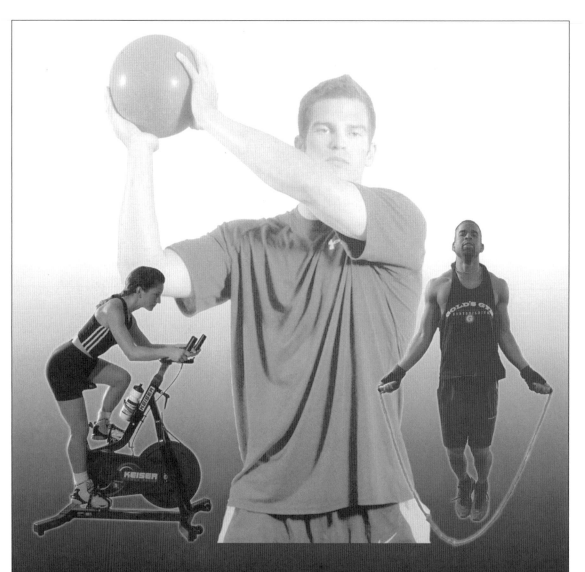

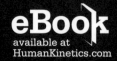